Start where you are.
Feel your way through.
Mistakes feed the soul. Char it well.

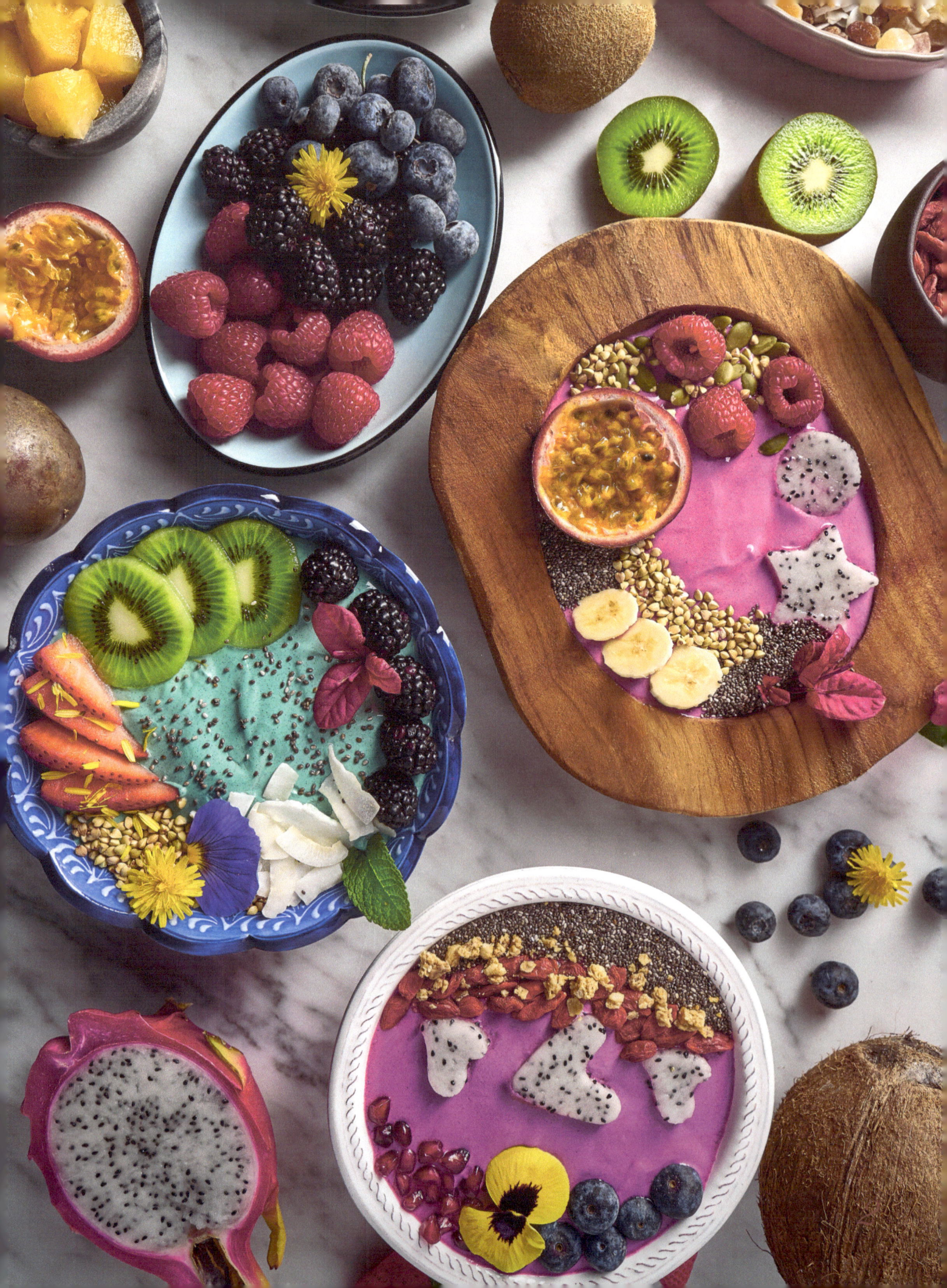

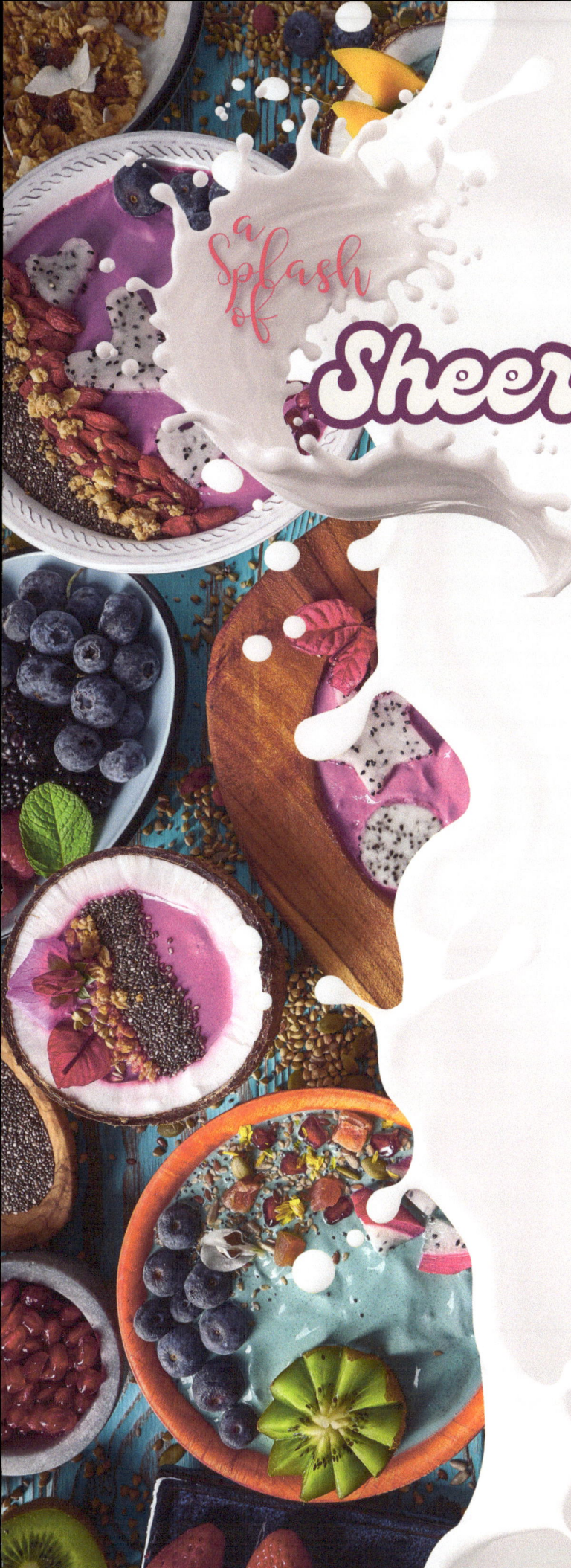

a Splash of Sheer

In my native language, sheer means milk, and this book is all about being sheer clear when it comes to revealing your true self. It focuses on making choices that are uniquely yours, recognizing the strength within you, and understanding the true essence of health.

Milk is the purest food and the first sustenance any child receives at the beginning of life. While this book may not be as pure as milk, it aims to guide you toward that purity. Each chapter will demonstrate just how sheer you can be!

Every chapter delves into different aspects of embracing your authentic self, encouraging you to strip away layers of doubt and external expectations. You'll find guidance on making decisions that resonate with your core values, discovering the power that lies within when you are truly aligned with your own truth. Health, both mental and physical, is addressed as an integral part of this journey, illustrating how clarity in self-awareness can lead to a more balanced and fulfilling life.

As you progress through the book, you'll encounter heartfelt stories and practical exercises designed to help you tap into your innate potential. By the end, you'll have a deeper understanding of what it means to live "sheer clear," equipped with the tools to embark on a transformative path toward authenticity. So, prepare to uncover the layers and step into the most genuine version of yourself, with the wisdom and clarity that this journey promises to bring.

ISBN: 979-8-9935592-1-6

Published by Papercast Industries
www.lulucure.com

Cover Design & Illustrations
Created by *Saleha Bukhari* using Canva Pro.
Select licensed elements were incorporated into original compositions; rights to third-party assets remain with their respective owners.

General Disclaimer
This book is created for educational and informational purposes only. It is not intended as a substitute for professional medical advice, diagnosis, or treatment. Readers should always consult a licensed healthcare provider before making health-related decisions. The author and publisher disclaim any liability for outcomes, injuries, or losses resulting from the application of the information contained herein.
This includes references to herbs, botanicals, lifestyle practices, natural materials, and holistic approaches to wellness. These are shared for inspiration and education, not as medical or therapeutic prescriptions. Readers are encouraged to seek professional guidance before adopting any wellness practices, especially if pregnant, nursing, taking medications, or managing chronic health conditions.

Cooking & Recipe Disclaimer
The recipes, techniques, and wellness practices shared in this book are offered for inspiration and education. Results may vary depending on ingredient quality, equipment, and individual skill. The author and publisher are not responsible for food allergies, dietary reactions, or adverse outcomes. Readers are urged to follow standard food safety practices, including proper handling, storage, and cooking temperatures, and to consult a qualified professional for any health or dietary concerns.

Credits & Acknowledgments
With deep gratitude to the Institute for Integrative Nutrition for shaping my understanding of holistic wellness. This work also draws upon research and insights from respected medical professionals and health organizations.
Above all, it is a tribute to the ancestral wisdom and lived experiences that continue to guide my journey, a lineage of nourishment, ritual, and resilience.

Edited & Designed by SALEHA BUKHARI

For my roots, my wings,
and the quiet voice that
said, "Keep going."

The Elements of Human Life: a Deeper Exploration

Throughout my journey in life, I have come to a profound understanding that the essence of being human is shaped by four interconnected elements: the body, the soul, feelings, and intelligence. At the heart of this intricate framework lie two primary components, the physical body and the soul, which together form the foundation of our existence. These core elements are further enriched by two secondary dimensions, where the body is intricately linked to our emotions and feelings, while the soul is deeply connected to our intellect and cognitive capabilities.

The body serves as our tangible, material connection to the world, embodying the experiences associated with earthly existence. It is a vessel that anchors us in the physical realm, demanding sustenance in the form of food, water, and care to sustain its vitality. Despite its temporal nature, the body plays a crucial role in our daily lives, influencing our interactions and perceptions as it grapples with the realities of aging, health, and mortality.

Feelings arise from our physical existence and can be seen as the heart of our emotional landscape. They are both a reflection of our bodily experiences and a powerful force that can guide our decisions. These emotions are not bound by logic; they instinctively respond to our desires, often leading us toward immediate gratification. However, this impulsive nature can also lead to regret if we are not mindful of their influence on our actions.

In contrast, the soul transcends the material world, connecting us to a deeper, more spiritual dimension of existence. It imbues our lives with meaning and purpose, providing a pathway to explore values, beliefs, and the essence of our being. The soul invites us to contemplate our place in the universe and encourages the pursuit of a higher understanding of life beyond the physical realm.

Intellect serves as the guiding force for the soul, channeling our thoughts and aspirations to facilitate wiser decision-making. It allows us to process our feelings critically, balancing desires with reason and foresight. By honoring our emotional experiences while employing rational thought, we can achieve lasting satisfaction and make choices that enhance our overall well-being.

Each of these elements complements the others, creating a unique display that defines the human experience. Every individual embodies a unique blend of these components, shaping their perspective, motivations, and interactions with the world. Understanding and nurturing each element can lead to a more harmonious existence as we strive to cultivate a balanced life that honors the intricate circle of our being.

How this Book Works:

In a world chasing artificial intelligence, this book is about something quieter and closer:
Living Intelligence.

The intelligence of food you cook yourself, habits you can trust, and seasons that teach you how to grow.

This is Volume One of a four-part collection. It's not a diet, not a quick fix; it's a companion. Whatever you bring here - joy, fatigue, chaos, or calm - these chapters are meant to feel like a hand in yours, guiding you back to steadiness and momentum.

Chapter One: Winter

The inward season. Rest, stabilize, reduce noise. Satiety-first meals and calming routines that make consistency easier.
Scope note: Structured guidance, not guarantees. Adjust pacing and portions to fit your body.

Chapter Two: Spring

The awakening season. Reconnect, brighten, build momentum. Clean, repeatable meal frameworks and metabolic steadiness that feel sustainable.
Scope note: Progress is personal. Adapt to your energy, schedule, and response.

Inside You'll Find

- <u>Mood maps</u> that meet you exactly where you are
- <u>Recipes as practice:</u> Cooking becomes a skill to learn, a way to discover health, and a source of joy in homemade meals
- <u>Micro-habits</u> that stack into lasting change
- <u>Reflections</u> to help you notice stress, boredom, or social pressure before they silence your Living Intelligence.

How to Begin

Start with the chapter that matches your energy.
Use the mood map when your day feels heavy or chaotic.
Cook, notice, adjust. Let the intelligence of small habits and steady meals guide you, while you keep living.

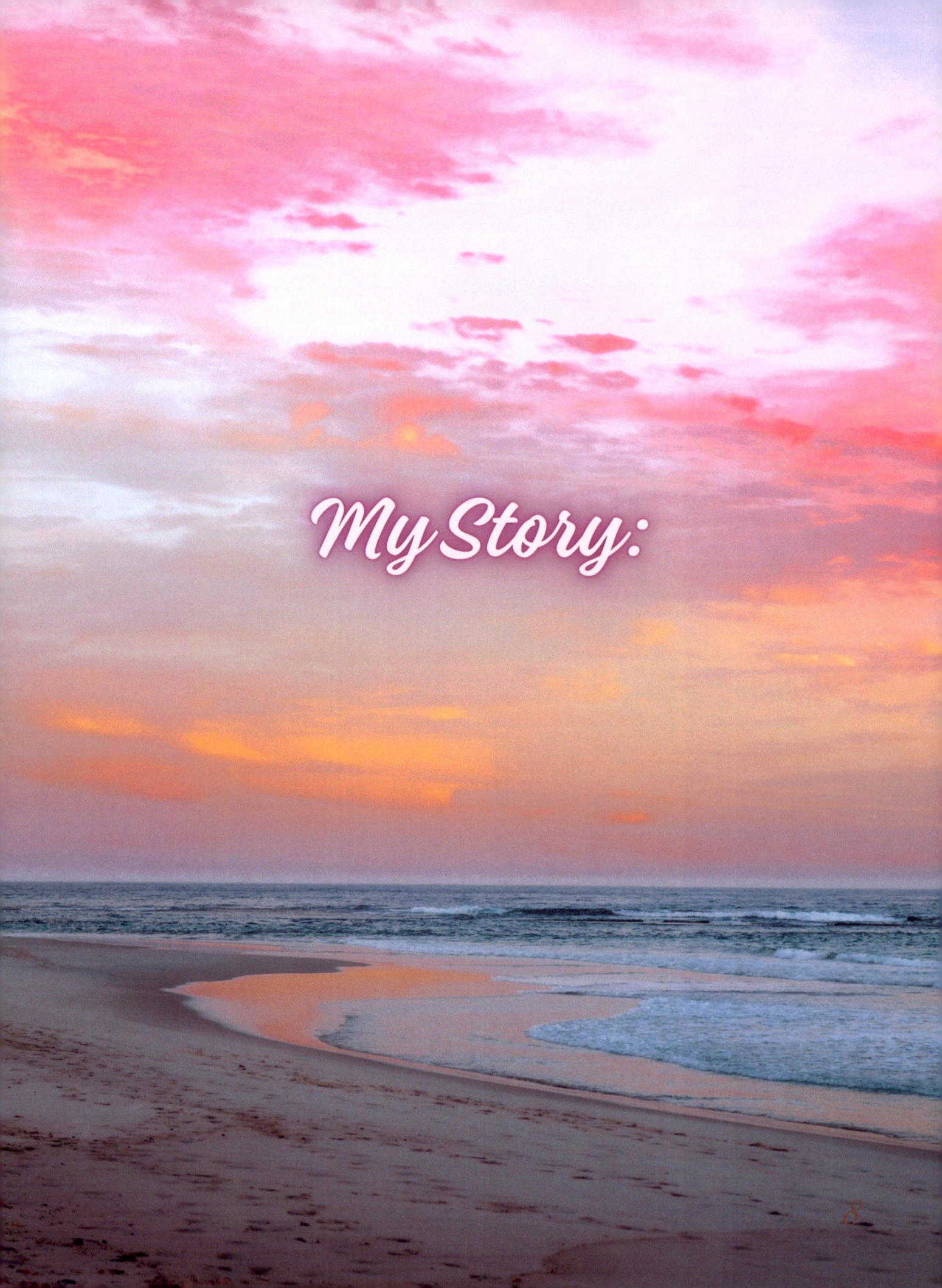

My Story:

"I will eat this meat raw!!" I remember the time my father unleashed those sharp words, his voice filled with frustration as he threw a bag of fresh meat across the kitchen, I was just eight years old, sitting cross-legged on a toashak (a long, cushioned mattress arrangement that adorned the floor of our living room, beautifully crafted by my mother). As I meticulously crocheted a colorful vest for myself and an equally vibrant one for the doll my mother had lovingly sewn for me, the atmosphere was punctuated with laughter as my siblings played nearby.

Suddenly, the serenity was shattered. I noticed my father, typically the embodiment of warmth and kindness, appearing distressed. He took his giant blood pressure pill, beads of sweat forming on his forehead, transforming his usually cheerful demeanor into one of noticeable anxiety. My siblings exchanged nervous glances, and while their fear was evident, my worry stemmed from the alarming presence of that pill—an object that signified something troubling. In that moment, a wave of intuition washed over me: I knew this wasn't right, that it was detrimental to my father's health. Without hesitation, I found my mother and approached her gently, my words laced with a hint of concern: "Please don't stress my dad!"

From that day forward, I began to associate health with emotional well-being. My father, the sweetest soul I had ever known, a gentle breeze of kindness and life, had lost his beloved mother during his teenage years. Growing up in a large family of ten siblings, I held a unique significance in his life as the first grandchild born to a son. This privilege was underscored by the fact that my father honored me by naming me after his mother, reinforcing my sense of belonging within his family. I often felt an unspoken bond that set me apart.

I was fortunate to grow up in a bilingual home, enriched by the influences of a third language, all while being enveloped in an atmosphere of love and vibrant cultural traditions. Yet, despite the warmth that surrounded us, life threw us some serious challenges to navigate as a family, often with limited resources.

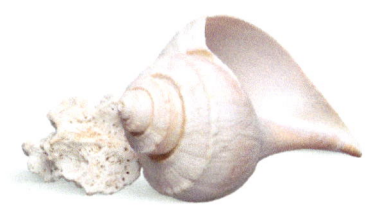
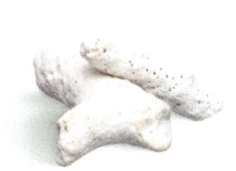

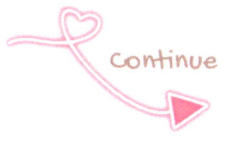
Continue

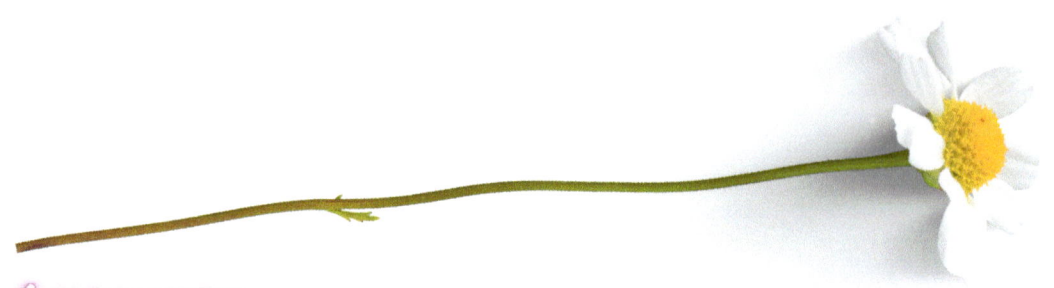

Long ago, my grandparents were forcibly uprooted from their homeland in Uzbekistan and sought refuge in Afghanistan. There, they embraced a new culture, learned Farsi, and adapted to a different way of life. It was in this vibrant yet demanding environment where my father pursued his college education to become a talented architect, while my mother flourished in her role as a homemaker. With a heart full of creativity, she mastered the art of culinary delights, transforming traditional recipes from Uzbekistan to incorporate local ingredients and flavors.

Their love story unfolded against this tapestry of resilience, and from this union, I was born—a blonde little girl cherished and adored by family and friends alike. However, the presence of war loomed large, forcing our family to leave behind everything we knew: our home, our memories, and the life we had built. This disturbance led us to Jeddah, a charming coastal city in Saudi Arabia, where the beauty of the landscape was overshadowed by my feelings of alienation. In this new home, my mother tirelessly dedicated herself to raising me and my siblings, instilling in us the values of uniqueness and independence, while my father provided us with love, comfort, and stability through his successful career.

Yet, after years of settling into this life, a new opportunity arose: the chance to move to the United States for higher education and to reconnect with extended family. This transition marked another significant shift, introducing me to a fresh environment, a new language, and a lifestyle packed with possibilities. Surrounded by warmth and acceptance, I quickly fell in love with the four distinct seasons that characterized my new home. I began to plant my roots here, feeling an increasing sense of belonging. Though I felt the weight of the pieces I had left behind, I still managed to carve out a sense of home in this new town.

As life continued to unfold around me, I found myself transforming in ways I never anticipated. I developed aspects of my personality that prioritized the expectations of others over my own needs, gradually distancing myself from the person I once was. In this process, I barely recognized my former self, and reclaiming that identity felt nearly impossible.

Instead of aligning my actions with my true self, I was only forging a path for existence, a path that was devoid of understanding my own needs and desires. This neglect left deep emotional scars and a significant toll on my health and ultimately resulting in significant weight gain. This change in my body was not just a number on a scale; it symbolized the disconnect between who I was and who I was trying to be.

I became severely anemic, constantly battling fatigue and weakness. Hormonal imbalances led to complications with my thyroid, further complicating my condition. I faced the frightening possibility of losing sight in one eye, an event that brought with it a wave of anxiety over my well-being. I also made the heart-wrenching decision to undergo surgery that resulted in the loss of an ovary, a choice that felt like surrendering a part of my identity.

The physical changes were accompanied by the unwelcome arrival of deep wrinkles, reminders of stress and neglect. My sense of purpose seemed to dissipate, leaving me adrift—a self-destructive machine operating without direction or care: it's amazing how moments can repeat themselves!

A defining moment arose when my children gathered around me, their little faces radiating concern as they expressed their heartfelt wish for my happiness and well-being. All they wished from me was to see me smile. Their words struck a chord deep within me, igniting a desire for change. I started a journey to redefine my life and discovered my passion for becoming a health coach. Initially, my goal was to heal my own well-being, but as I navigated this path of personal growth, I found myself gaining clarity and direction in my world. It was as if I had been reborn, full of energy and optimism, ready to embrace what life had to offer. This unexpected twist of fate allowed my past experiences to intertwine with who I am today, unveiling new opportunities and perspectives. The challenges I had faced became invaluable lessons that shaped my character and resilience. Through this journey, my mission became crystal clear: to share my experiences and insights with other souls who might resonate with my struggles.

This book is a beacon of hope for everyone who shine brightly in a crowd and rise above challenges! it's an inspiration for those eager to ignite their inner brilliance. It speaks to every wondering soul in search of a genuine sense of belonging, to individuals who have confronted the cruelty of bullying, every person grappling with self-doubt regarding their significance, It's to honor mothers who have bravely navigated the wild waves of body changes to bring new life.
For those who shattered the mold to grow wild and whole.
This book belongs to you. To us. To anyone ready to step into their light.

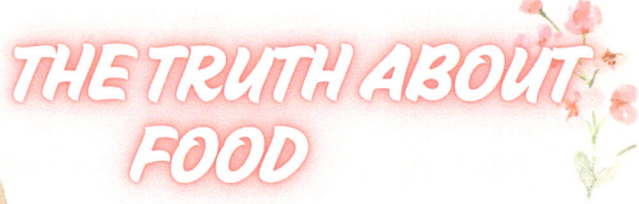

THE TRUTH ABOUT FOOD

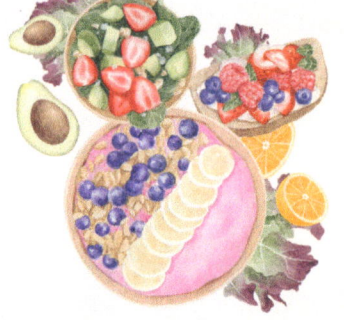

We nourish the body, but true sustenance is something else entirely. Food, as we know it, is a custom of survival, a necessity, a fleeting satisfaction. But beyond the plate, beyond the bite, beyond the hunger that rises and falls, there is a deeper kind of feeding.

Think of the cake, not just as sugar and flour, but as a vessel of memory. As children, it was never just the sweetness that brought joy.

It was the laughter at the table, the hands that passed the plate, the presence of those who loved us. Years later, when we taste that same cake, it is not the ingredients that warm us, it is the echo of those moments, the ghosts of old happiness returning for one brief, beautiful visit.

We consume meals, but we feast on connection. We drink in the words of a mentor, devour the thrill of discovery, inhale the quiet understanding found in another's eyes. These are the elements that truly fill us—the kind that cannot be prepared in a kitchen or served on a tray.

Food, in the traditional sense, will sustain us for a day. But what of the nourishment that lasts a lifetime? The love that fortifies us, the dreams that propel us, the wisdom that becomes part of our very being? This is the true feast, the one that does not perish, does not spoil, does not fade.

So, let us eat. But more than that, let us be fed by life itself, by the unseen, the untasted, the immeasurable forces that shape us into who we are. For it is not the bread that sustains us, but the beauty of the hands that break it.

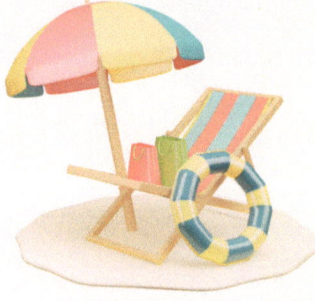

IN this flavorful exploration, I will share valuable insight into the deeper meanings of food in our lives. Across four thoughtfully crafted chapters, I invite you to discover the small yet significant gifts that true food can offer us, unveiling its true sheer essence.

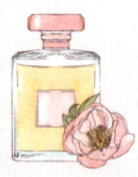

Additionally, I will delight your palate with delicious home-cooked recipes that will not only satisfy your taste buds but also enrich your overall food experience.

Join me in uncovering the true nature of food; an exploration that celebrates its role as both nourishment and a profound expression of identity and connection.

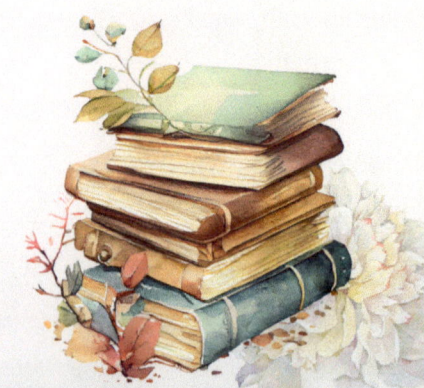

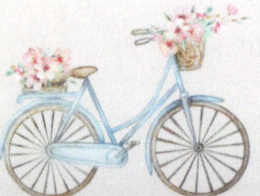

EACH PAGE of this book resonates with its own unique rhythm, capturing the essence of individual moments through carefully selected colors that inspire specific feelings. Each recipe is infused with personal significance, reflecting the emotions and experiences that shaped my journey. Every element within these pages has a distinct soul, contributing to the narrative of my life over the years. As you turn each page, let the textures, scents, and flavors leap out to greet you. This book isn't just a recipe collection; it's my heart speaking through life and culinary tales, crafted over a year of passion and introspection. If you feel that my voice is not present in some pages, you will definitely find me expressed through the inspiring imagery and thoughtful elements that accompany **EACH PAGE.**

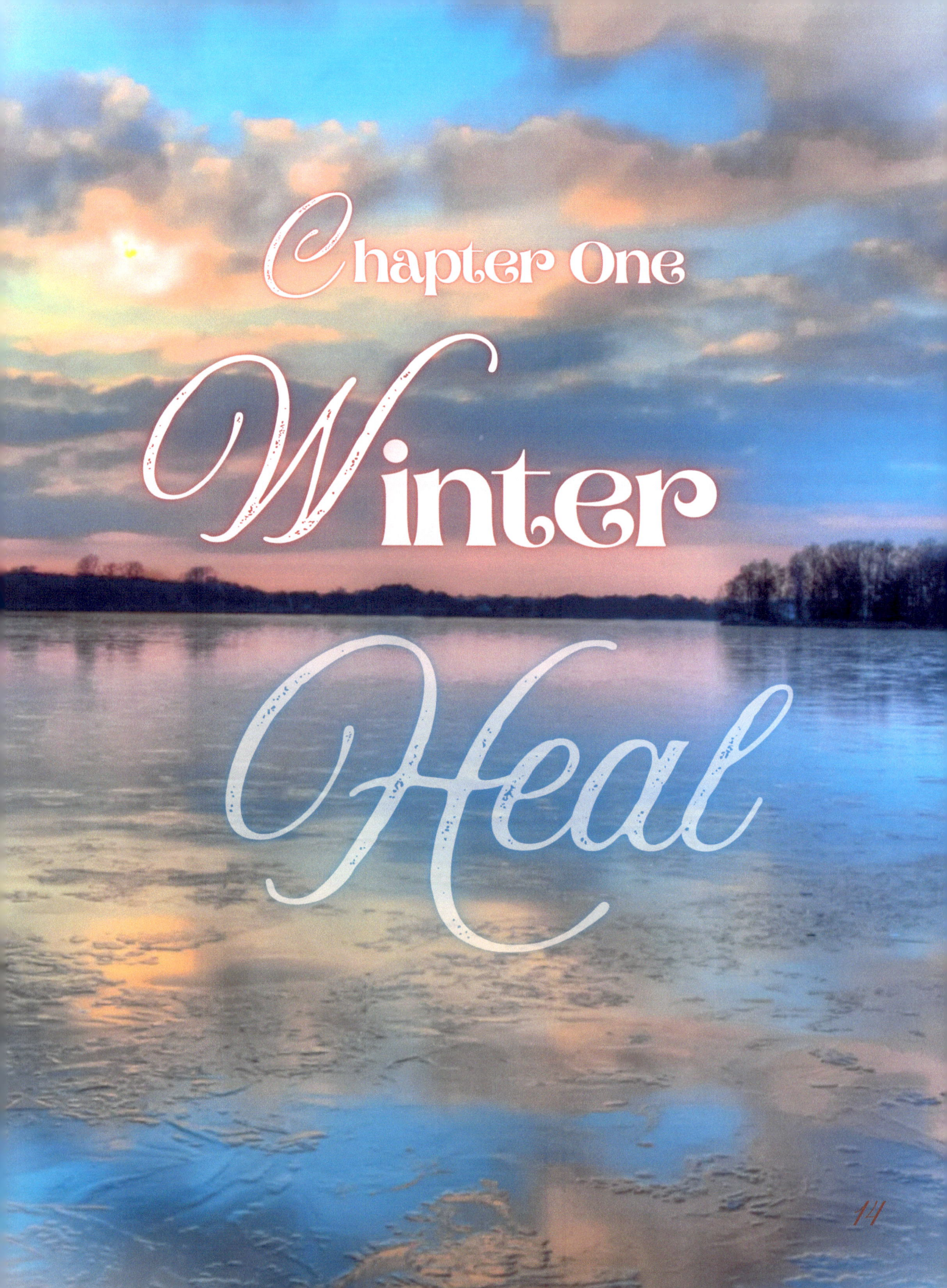

Chapter One

Winter

Heal

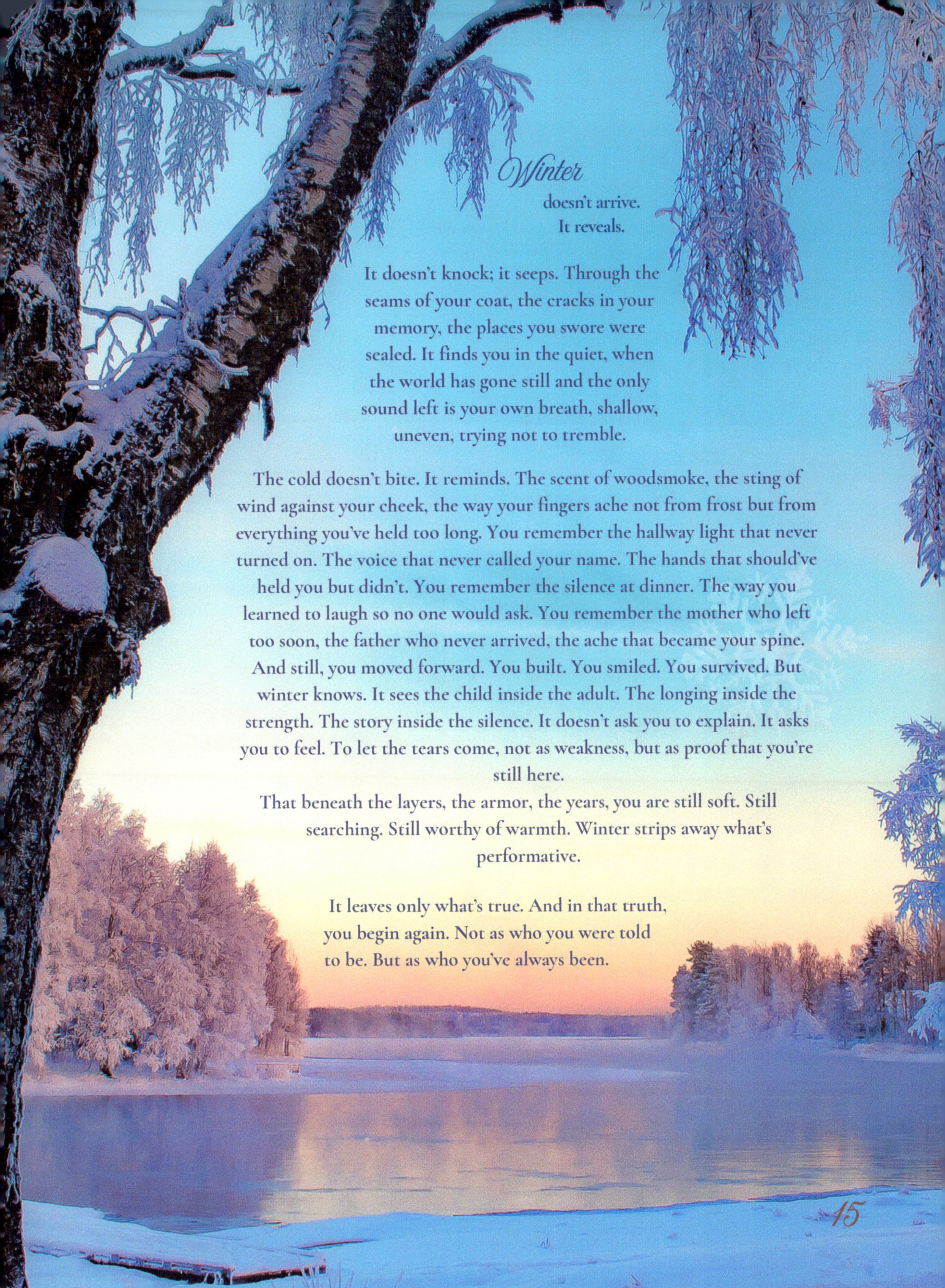

Winter

doesn't arrive.
It reveals.

It doesn't knock; it seeps. Through the seams of your coat, the cracks in your memory, the places you swore were sealed. It finds you in the quiet, when the world has gone still and the only sound left is your own breath, shallow, uneven, trying not to tremble.

The cold doesn't bite. It reminds. The scent of woodsmoke, the sting of wind against your cheek, the way your fingers ache not from frost but from everything you've held too long. You remember the hallway light that never turned on. The voice that never called your name. The hands that should've held you but didn't. You remember the silence at dinner. The way you learned to laugh so no one would ask. You remember the mother who left too soon, the father who never arrived, the ache that became your spine. And still, you moved forward. You built. You smiled. You survived. But winter knows. It sees the child inside the adult. The longing inside the strength. The story inside the silence. It doesn't ask you to explain. It asks you to feel. To let the tears come, not as weakness, but as proof that you're still here.

That beneath the layers, the armor, the years, you are still soft. Still searching. Still worthy of warmth. Winter strips away what's performative.

It leaves only what's true. And in that truth, you begin again. Not as who you were told to be. But as who you've always been.

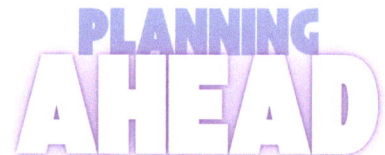

PLANNING AHEAD

Planning isn't about perfection. It's about presence.
It's how chaos gets a container. How scattered
thoughts start to make sense.
I start with paper. Not because it's cute.
Because it's real.
The weight of a notebook. The grip of a pen.
They remind me: this matters.

Some days, I want clean lines and quiet pages.
Other days, I need color, texture, attitude.
My tools match my mood.
They hold my thoughts without judgment.

Receipts? No.
The chemicals in them don't belong in
my bloodstream-or my ideas.

Inspiration doesn't wait.
It shows up in the cold, at the kitchen
counter, mid-errand.
So I stay ready.
Not perfect. Just ready.

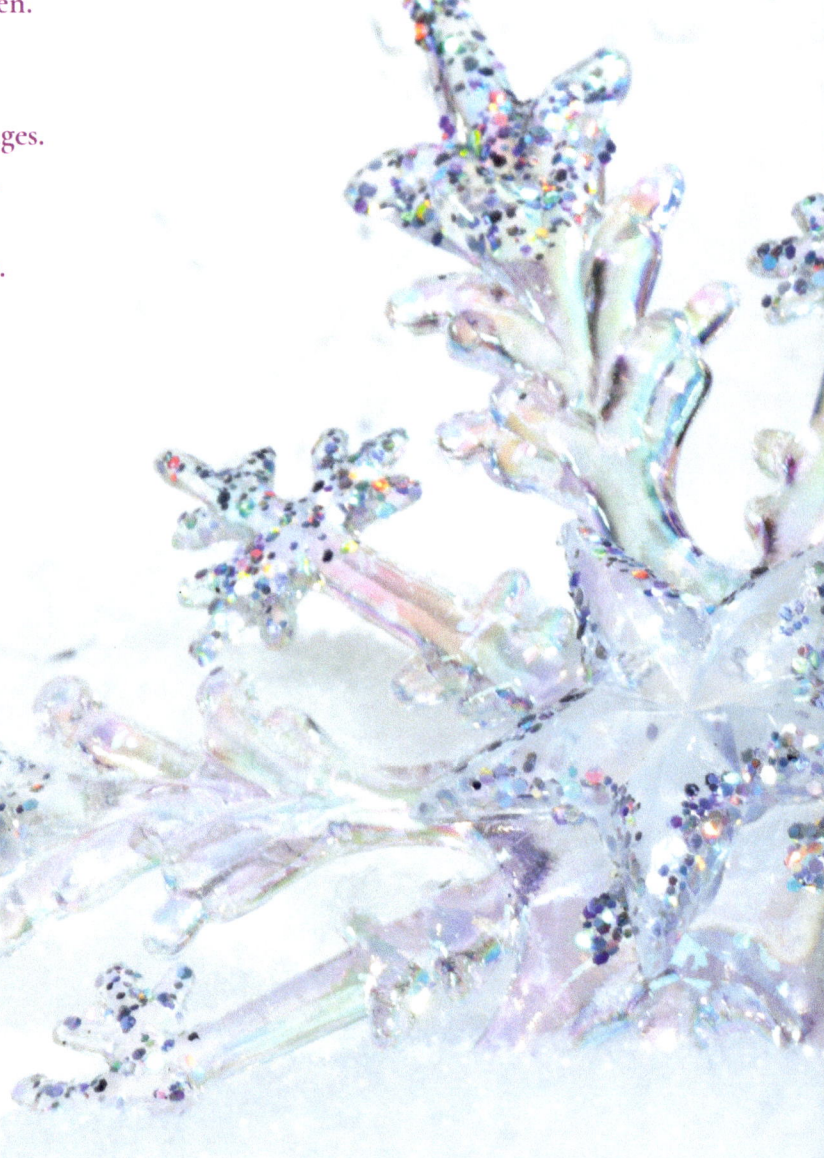

The best kind of
planning?
The kind
that lets your
thoughts breathe.
Let them spill. Let
them stretch.
They don't have to
make sense yet.

Because later-when the dust settles,
when the patterns emerge,
when the future starts to whisper- you'll be ready to answer.

Plan like you're building something sacred.
Plan like your legacy depends on it.
Because it does.

Planning

Throughout this chapter, I'll share weekly strategies designed to help you connect with the most authentic version of yourself. But here's the thing: these methods aren't meant to be followed rigidly. They are meant to be felt, adapted, infused with your own spirit. Because the most powerful planning is the kind that truly belongs to you.

Along the way, I'll sprinkle in some affirmations and thoughts, gentle nudges to realign your intentions, quiet reminders that bring clarity when life feels scattered. These words aren't here to tell you what to do, but rather to help you see yourself more clearly, to guide you toward a planning journey that feels meaningful, effortless, and deeply personal.

So, step into this space. Let it be fluid, flexible, uniquely yours.
Because the secret
to fulfillment isn't
in the structure
itself, it's in the way
you make it
your own.

PLANNING *MONDAY*

1- *Hair Love Ritual:* Let your hair drink in some nourishment. Whether it's a rich mask, a warm oil treatment, or just giving your scalp a little extra attention, let this be a reset. Damp strands, a generous coat of argan or coconut oil, and a moment to let it soak in, restoring the softness you deserve.

2- *Fridge Revival:* Out with the old, in with the fresh! Time to clear the leftovers that have overstayed their welcome. A quick wipe-down with a vinegar-water solution and suddenly, your fridge feels lighter, cleaner, and ready for new possibilities. Maybe even sneak in a snack afterward; you've earned it.

3- *Meal Magic Prep:* Pick a meal that excites you for next Monday. Something cozy, something vibrant, something that makes you look forward to the week ahead. Jot down the ingredients, make it smooth and effortless. The best meals are the ones planned with a little love.

4- *Mindful Start:* Before the week fully takes hold, pause. One deep breath, one quiet thought, one small act of kindness toward yourself. A cup of something warm, a stretch, a journal page, or simply stillness. Mondays can be gentle too.

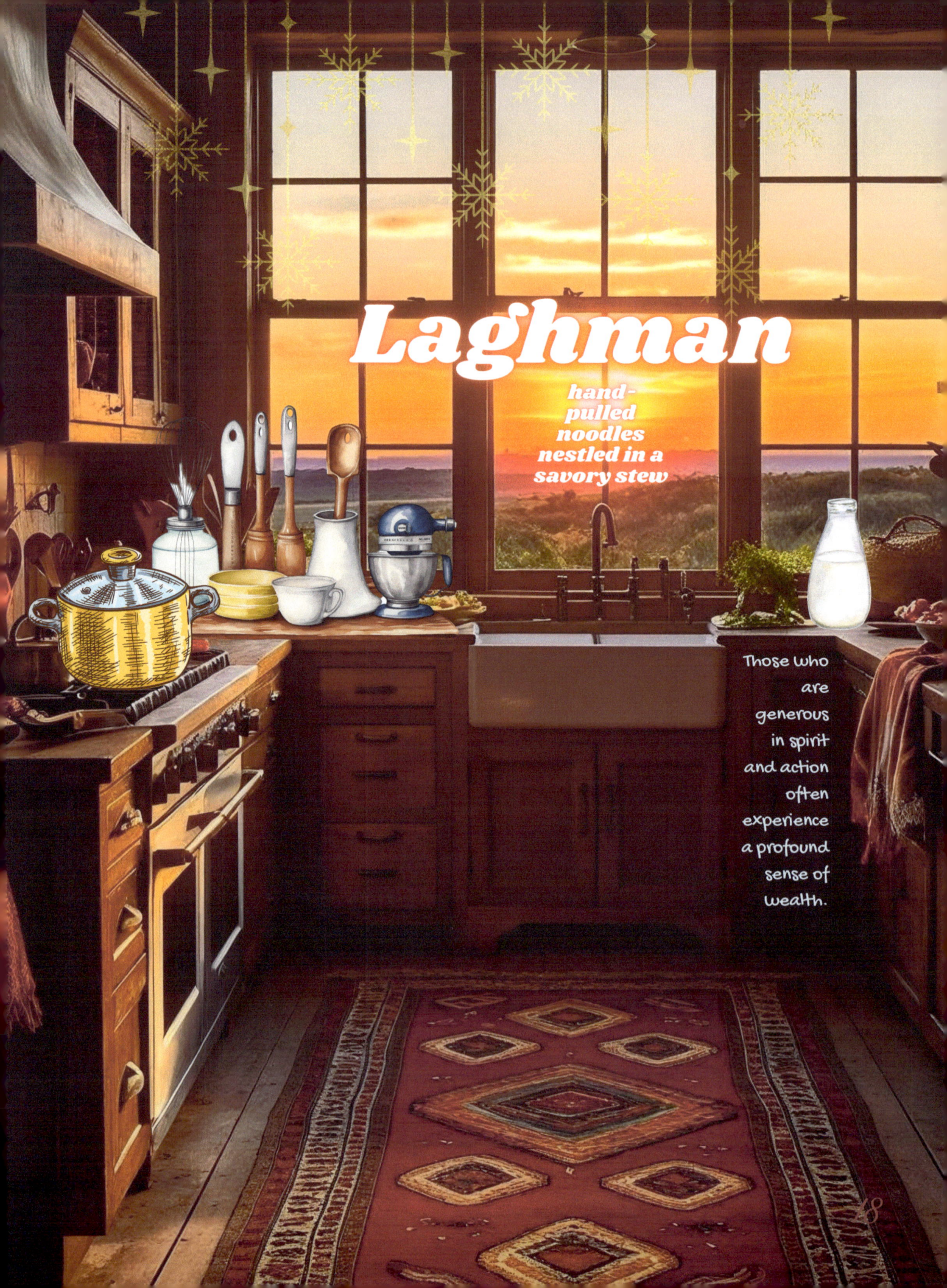

Laghman

hand-pulled noodles nestled in a savory stew

Those who are generous in spirit and action often experience a profound sense of wealth.

The connection I have with Laghman goes beyond bare memory; it represents a lifelong relationship steeped in tradition. This bond began in second grade when my mother first invited me into the warmth of our kitchen. I distinctly remember being tasked with cutting vegetables, a seemingly simple activity that proved to be challenging at first. My early attempts at slicing green beans were far from impressive; I struggled with control and technique. Yet, my mother, embodying both patience and wisdom, gently guided my hands, demonstrating how to achieve the perfect angle for slicing. Through these moments, she instilled in me the understanding that cooking transcends following a recipe; it is also a form of art that involves creativity, intuition, and a personal touch.

Cooking, she taught me, is not just about following instructions. It's an art, a dance between intuition and technique, a reflection of the heart.

That lesson never left me. Over the years, Laghman became my canvas; each spice, each twist in the recipe carrying its own expression, its own moment of discovery. Some days, I honored tradition. Other days, I let creativity take the lead. Every modification deepened the bond, turning a simple meal into a piece of me.

If I were to give Laghman a name beyond its own, I would call it Marriage. Not for love alone, but for the intricate balance it demands, the blending of flavors, the harmony of textures, the quiet understanding that each ingredient has a role to play. Some elements require patience. Some ask for precision. Some thrive in contrast, others in perfect unity.

Nothing in Laghman exists by accident. The vegetables, handpicked, cut not just for size but for balance. The protein, chosen with care, meant to nourish, to satisfy. The noodles, handmade, stretched, shaped, their very existence a labor of love.

And then comes the moment, the first twirl of noodles, the first taste. The flavors don't just land; they waltz, weaving through the senses, whispering: Live it fully. Every bite, every breath, every moment.

Sharing Laghman with loved ones is magic. It turns simple conversation into something richer, turns laughter into something warmer. It has the power to bring people home, whether home is a place, a memory, or simply the comfort found in one another.

It isn't just food. It's a hug, a piece of history, a silent embrace from the generations that came before. Laghman carries stories: of family, of resilience, of connection. It is rich and grounding, a bowl of warmth when life feels too cold, an invitation to slow down, to savor, to belong.

And if there's one quiet truth hidden in every bite, it's this:

Life, much like Laghman, is built in layers. Some moments are bold, bursting with flavor. Others are quiet, subtle, woven delicately into the background. Some require time, patience, care, the willingness to let things unfold as they should.

Nothing worth savoring is rushed.

So twirl your fork, take the bite, let the warmth settle in. And remember, the best things in life take time, love, and a touch of faith in the process.

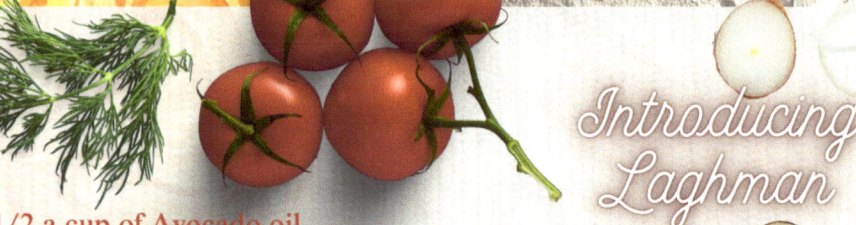

Introducing Laghman

1/2 a cup of Avocado oil

1 tbsp Ghee (Using ghee will elevate the unique flavor in this dish, instead of traditional animal fat.)

1 Onion cut into thin slices

1 pound of Flank steak or chuck steak cut into half-inch cubes (or portobello mushrooms to replace)

Salt and pepper (This dish is a true masterpiece as it manages to deliver a delightful burst of flavors while utilizing only a modest amount of spices. The process of preparing it correctly is key in achieving a profound and exquisite taste.)

3 tbsp Garlic, minced

3-4 Tomatoes (If you can get your hands on some locally sourced organic ingredients, you're in for a real treat! Trust me, your Laghman will be absolutely delicious.)

3 tbsp of Tomato paste

2 tsp Organic Vegetable Bouillon paste

3 Bay leaves

4 cups of Water

1 small Eggplant, cut into 1-inch cubes.

1/2 pound Brussels sprouts: "To make larger pieces more edible, cut them into halves or quarters."

1 Potatoes "Cut into small one-inch cubes"

1 cup Green beans "Cut at an angle into small pieces."

2 Carrots "Cut into cubes that are half an inch in size."

2 stalks Celery

1 cup Cabbage "shredded"

Handful of fresh Dill (optional)

"Use organic ingredients when possible for a cleaner, more honest flavor."

> Once you've made it a few times, you'll find yourself tossing in the ingredients by instinct, no measuring needed. That's when you'll know you've truly mastered the recipe.

Freezing Tip: (4-6 months)

When I'm chopping up veggies, I like to think ahead! I double my usual amount, wash and prep the extras, and then stash them away in airtight bags or containers. It's a great way to save time and ensure I have healthy ingredients ready to go whenever I need them! Plus, there's something satisfying about having a little stash in the freezer just waiting for a delicious meal.

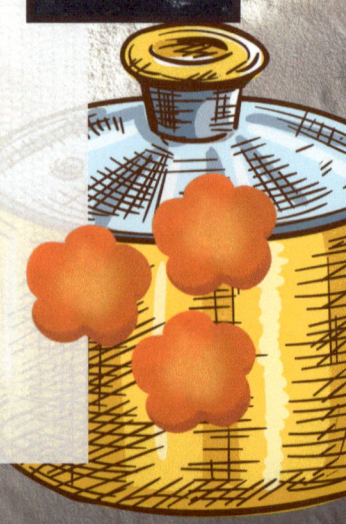

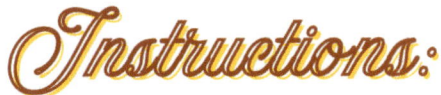

Instructions:

1- To make this dish, you first need to heat up a large stainless-steel pan. Once the pan is heated, add oil and ghee before adding the onions. Make sure that you stir the onions well and then turn down the heat to a low setting. Cover the pan to allow the onions to steam and become transparent. When the onions are ready, remove the lid and turn up the heat. As this dish is based on onions, it is important that they are caramelized to perfection. Take a good look at the onions and smell them. The ideal color should be dark tan, but not brown. You will know that the onions are ready when they have developed a beautiful caramelized flavor and color.

2- Get ready to add the star of your dish - the meat! This is where you turn up the heat, and let the magic happen. Make sure to season the meat with salt and pepper and stir continuously on high heat. Although it may get a little hot, don't worry - you can wear mittens to protect your hands. Make sure to choose the correct spatula for this process - a long-handled round spatula with a flat tip is perfect. As you stir, take in the aroma, and enjoy the cooking process. Wait until your meat is beautifully browned and let it develop a deep flavor without the need for additional enhancements. Add garlic and stir for a minute. Now it's time to add the tomatoes! Remember to cut them into small pieces instead of pureeing them. This simple tip will help you achieve the perfect balance of sweetness and tang.

3- Lower the heat of your pan and cover it with a lid. Let the tomato cook for about two minutes. Once done, turn up the heat to high and stir constantly until you hear a sizzling sound, indicating that all the liquid from the tomato has evaporated. Add the tomato paste and stir for another minute. Be vigilant and make sure the bottom of the pan does not get too sticky or brown, or else the tomato will burn. It's time to add water, bay leaf, and bouillon. Let the mixture boil before adding in the eggplant. Lower the heat to medium-low and let everything cook for 30-45 minutes until the eggplant falls apart. The base sauce is now done.

4- While your sauce is cooking, make the noodles.

5- Preparing meals can be a time-consuming task, and having to make the base sauce every time you cook can add to the workload. However, with a little bit of planning, you can save yourself a lot of time and effort in the kitchen. Why not make the sauce a day or two in advance and keep it refrigerated? Alternatively, you can freeze it once it's cooled down and have it ready for use whenever you need it! This way, you'll be able to focus on enjoying your meals without having to worry about the prep work.

6- Now, it's time to add color and fun to the meat! Start with potatoes, brussels sprouts, and green beans, let it boil on medium-low for 7 minutes.

Continue

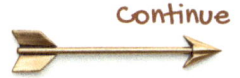

21

7- Place the cooked noodles into a generously sized personal pasta bowl.

8- Remove the lid and take a deep breath to inhale the aroma of the delicious dish you've prepared! Admire the vibrant colors and feel grateful for the ability to enjoy simple pleasures in life. Give the meat sauce a quick stir and pour approximately two cups of it over the noodles using a soup spatula. Sprinkle some chopped dill on top for garnish and serve.

9- Indulge in the delectable taste of Laghman, traditionally paired with lemon or vinegar and laza. The sauce itself is so rich in flavor that it encapsulates the full experience in a single bite.

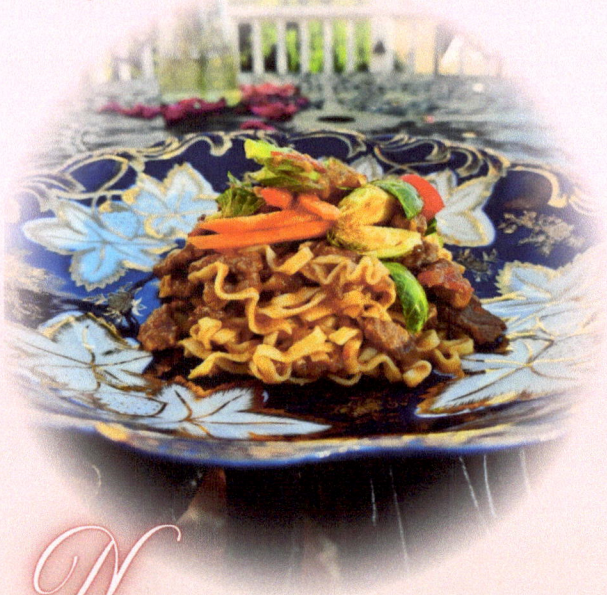

Cooking is not just about following a recipe; it's a way of creating a unique and inspiring experience. When you connect emotionally with the process, you infuse each step with your own energy and feelings. So when the meal is ready, it's not just a reward, it's a pile of love (or hate in some cases) that can heal your emotional wounds or express gratitude. Master the art of cooking and enjoy Laghman with tears of joy or tears of letting go

Notes

- Cooking vegetables requires precise timing to achieve the right texture and flavor.
- Eggplant should be cooked the longest until it falls apart for sauces.
- Potatoes should be cooked for about 10 minutes to avoid falling apart and affecting texture.
- Brussels sprouts and green beans should be cooked until soft but not mushy.
- Carrots and celery should be cooked briefly to retain crunchiness.
- Cabbage should be added at the end of cooking to maintain a crunchy texture and avoid overcooking.

Gym Reflections

To promote understanding among diverse communities, it is equally essential to nurture the powerful virtue of forgiveness. Much like how we hone our physical abilities, whether it's the graceful act of walking, the precise skill of driving, or the melodic mastery of playing an instrument, through consistent practice, we can likewise cultivate the habit of forgiveness through intentional and mindful engagement.

This process involves seeking out moments that challenge us to forgive, deeply reflecting on our emotions, and consciously making the choice to release our grievances and heal from past hurts. By doing so, we open ourselves up to personal growth and foster stronger connections with others.

January:
The Gossip Season

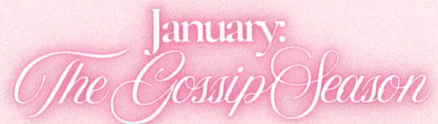

January, the month where gossip thrives, slithering through conversations like smoke curling from a villain's cigar. The world outside is frozen, bare, silent. And in that silence? The whispers grow louder.

People sit in cafés, coats pulled tight, exchanging glances that say Tell me everything. Texts fly— Did you hear? Can you believe? What were they thinking? There's something almost delicious about the drama, like feeding off the cold, turning isolation into a game, a spectacle, a stage.

It starts innocently. A comment, an opinion, a well-placed I just find it interesting that... But soon, it morphs. Sides are taken. Stories stretch. Truth bends. And somewhere in the chaos, someone is left out in the cold, wondering how they became the villain of a tale they never agreed to be in.

But here's the thing, gossip is a fragile kind of power. It builds quickly, but it crumbles just as fast. A single act of kindness, a moment of understanding, has the power to burn through it like sunlight melting snow.

Because warmth in winter doesn't just come from fireplaces and heavy coats, it comes from people choosing to make the world softer, brighter, more whole. The ones who visit an old friend in need, show up at shelters with hands open instead of folded in judgment, give their time not because they have to, but because they understand what it means to be seen.

Laughter—real laughter, the kind that comes from joy, not judgment, shifts the story. A warm invitation, a moment of shared understanding, a choice to pull someone in instead of casting them out... this is the redemption arc of winter.

So yes, revel in the drama for a moment. Take your sip of intrigue, let the villainous grin spread, feel the thrill of the whisper. And then.... choose better.

Rewrite the season.

Let January be the month where warmth wins, where connection deepens, where kindness steps forward like the unexpected hero of the story.

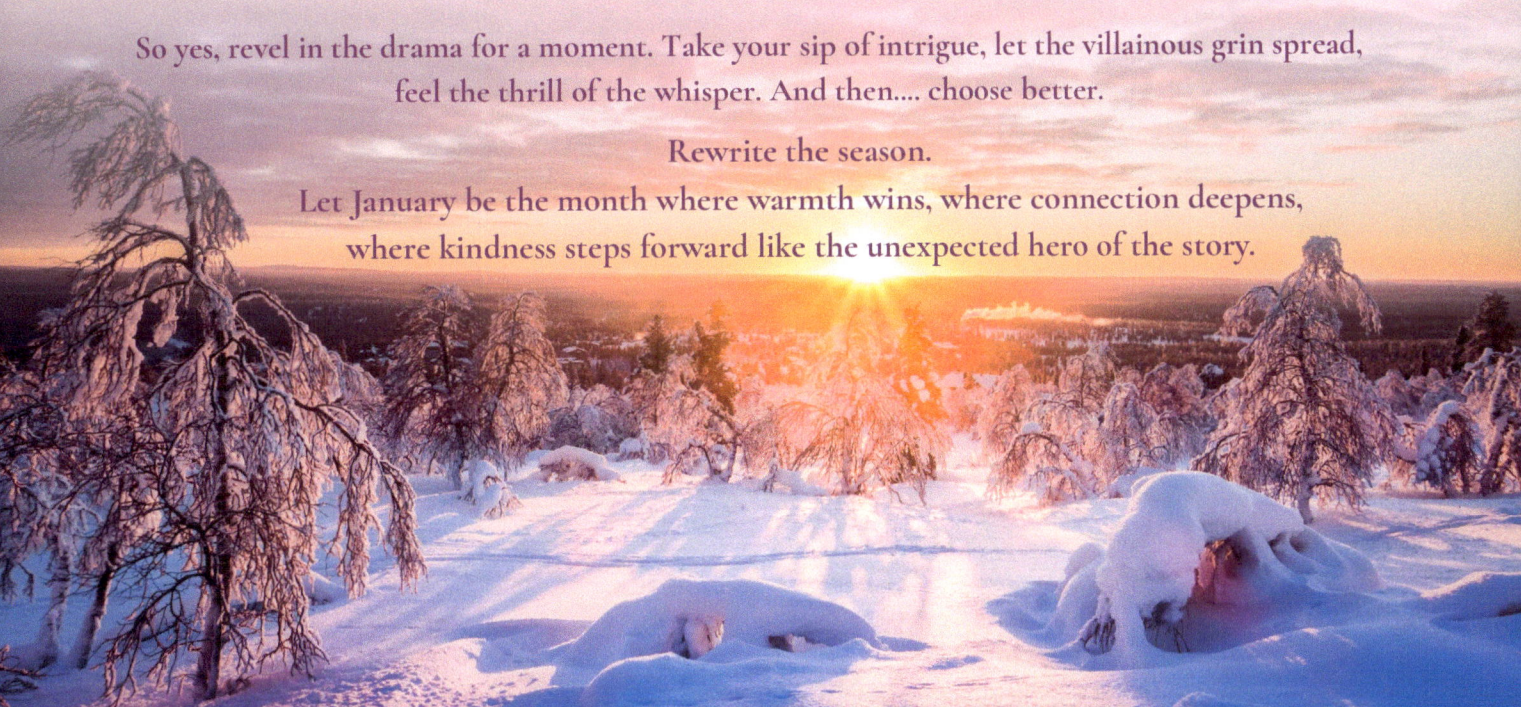

Affirmations

As winter settles in, it's easy to fall into a cozy trap of laziness and procrastination. The allure of warm blankets and hot drinks can lead to a growing mountain of unfinished tasks. Unfortunately, this often means that when the vibrant energy of spring arrives, we find ourselves scrambling to tackle a backlog of work that we know we could have handled with much more focus and effort. Rather than waiting for the thaw to kickstart our motivation, let's embrace the present moment and get things done now. Seize the day, make today the day you take action!

To Inspire you during these colder months, here are some affirmations to uplift your spirit and keep you on track:

1. I am here. Not halfway, not hidden. Here. Fully, fiercely, undeniably present in my own life.

2. I do not wait to feel ready; I trust myself now. The steps I take today shape the future I once only dreamed of.

3. The cold does not strip me; it strengthens me. Like fire forging steel, every challenge shapes me into something unbreakable.

4. I am not lost; I am evolving. Every small choice, every quiet moment is proof that I am building myself into something powerful.

5. I do not abandon myself. I move at my own rhythm. I listen, I grow, I rise. In this, I claim my strength.

I do not break. I do not disappear. I remain. And that is enough.

Aging gracefully is a journey embraced by many confident individuals, yet when this journey leads you down the path of insulin resistance (IR), the experience can become more challenging than beautiful. The elegance of wrinkles, symbols of the wisdom and respect acquired over the years, loses its charm when accompanied by the visible effects of IR.

Instead of embodying the gracefulness that comes with age, one may face an unhealthy appearance characterized by sagging skin, unsightly skin tags, and hyperpigmentation in certain areas. Perhaps the most undesirable consequence is the notorious "muffin top," a byproduct of weight gain and hormonal changes that can accompany insulin resistance. These conditions can contribute to a sense of discomfort and a diminished self-image, creating an inner struggle while facing the external signs of aging.

Insulin resistance is a multifaceted condition influenced by a combination of factors. Its origins often stem from a complex interplay of unhealthy dietary choices, such as a diet predominantly high in refined sugars and trans fats, alongside a lifestyle characterized by insufficient physical activity. Sedentary habits prevalent in modern life exacerbate this condition. Additionally, genetic predispositions can increase susceptibility, with some individuals inheriting a higher likelihood of developing metabolic dysfunctions. To effectively treat insulin resistance, it is vital to comprehend its root causes. Individuals seeking to mitigate its effects can adopt informed dietary strategies that prioritize the consumption of whole, nutrient-dense foods. A diet rich in fresh fruits, vibrant vegetables, lean sources of protein, and whole grains supports metabolic health and aids in weight management. Furthermore, incorporating consistent physical activity into daily routines, whether through aerobic exercises, strength training, or recreational activities, can significantly improve insulin sensitivity and overall well-being.

By addressing these factors, individuals can reclaim their vitality and establish a foundation for graceful aging, maintaining both physical well-being and a youthful spirit.

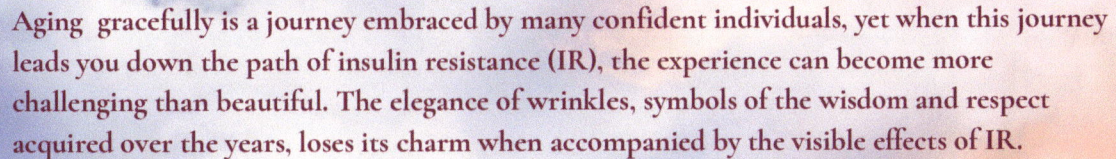

Insulin Resistance: A Glimpse at Aging With Grace

Laza

Peeled Organic Garlic
(6 oz Bag)

1/2
a cup of
Pepper Flakes

1 cup of
Great
Quality
Olive Oil

1 TSP
Cayenne
Pepper

The traditional way to enjoy Laghman is by complementing it with a tangy element, such as fresh lemon juice or a splash of vinegar, along with a generous helping of Laza. Laza is a delightful, homemade spicy chili sauce that brings an exhilarating burst of heat paired with a subtle, garlicky undertone, transforming your Laghman experience to a whole new level of flavor. When I find myself running low on my homemade Laza, I often resort to store-bought sriracha sauce, which offers a decent kick. However, if you truly want to elevate your dish to a level 10 in both heat and depth of flavor, let's delve into the art of making Laza from scratch:

LET'S MAKE LAZA

1- Start by slicing peeled garlic into thin slivers. If time is short, simply throw the garlic in a small blender and roughly chop it until the pieces are mostly uniform.

2- Heat oil in a small saucepan for about a minute, then add the garlic. Let the garlic sizzle gently over low heat, taking care to stir occasionally, to prevent sticking. After 5-7 minutes, when the garlic turns a beautiful golden bronze and fills the kitchen with its aroma, remove it from the heat.

3- Stir in red pepper flakes and cayenne pepper, then let it cool. Store Laza in an airtight container in the fridge to enhance any pasta dish with love.

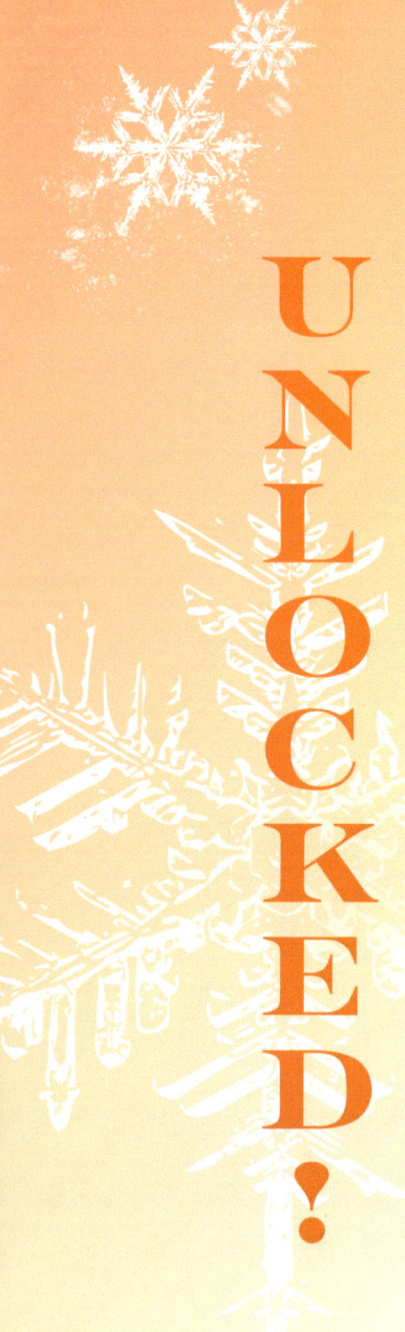

UNLOCKED!

There's something fascinating about joy, it's supposed to be effortless, magnetic, impossible to resist. Yet, I often find myself standing in the middle of a celebration, surrounded by laughter, conversations bouncing off the walls, the kind of electric energy that should make my soul dance, and somehow, I feel... detached. Not sad. Not lonely. Just a little out of sync, like I accidentally hit the "mute" button on my ability to enjoy the moment.

The culprit? Oh, it varies wildly. Sometimes it's stress piling up, an old disappointment lurking in the background, a whisper of heartbreak that hasn't fully faded—or, in true betrayal fashion, my morning coffee deciding to go cold before I get a single glorious sip.

But here's the surprising part, those moments of disconnection aren't just frustrating; they're actually secret windows into my own mind. Little clues left behind, waiting to be decoded. And when I pause long enough to examine them, they don't just dissolve, they reveal something about me, about the patterns I carry, about the way I've learned (and sometimes unlearned) joy. Growing up, my home was built on love; strong, undeniable, the kind of warmth that could be felt even in silence. But it was also built on caution, sprinkled with a healthy dose of 'be careful, don't risk too much' and 'let's think about all the possible disasters before we dive in.' My parents, wonderful and wise, had perfected the art of preparation, making sure I was ready for every curveball life might throw my way. And while I'm endlessly grateful for that wisdom, it did leave me with a tendency to anticipate the worst! sometimes before the worst was even remotely close to happening.

Fast forward to today, and I realize that, occasionally, my brain still operates like an overprotective coach, warning me to "not get too comfortable" with happiness in case it's fleeting. But the biggest lesson life has handed me is this: happiness isn't a trick—it's meant to be embraced.

So now, when I feel that disconnect creeping in, I don't let it take over. I shake it off. I laugh at my cold coffee betrayal. I remind myself that I deserve to be fully present in my own joy. Because life? It isn't some cautious, tiptoed journey, it's meant to be fully, shamelessly, gloriously lived.

Finding Freedom in Joy

There are moments when I catch myself in that familiar thought: I hate being here. The weight of routine, the sameness, the feeling of being stuck, it can all press so heavily against the soul. But I've learned something about escaping that mindset: sometimes, the best way to break free is to break a few rules, not recklessly, not harmfully, but in a way that reminds me life isn't just obligation and expectation.

For me, that might mean slipping into a boutique, eyeing a pair of breathtakingly expensive shoes, and deciding, without hesitation, that they belong to me. Not because I need them, but because they spark something. Because sometimes, joy isn't practical, it's impulsive, it's the thrill of doing something simply because it makes you feel alive.

But it isn't always about grand gestures. Sometimes, the real luxury is a pause, a moment to step outside the rush, to breathe deeply, to actually see the world around me. In the chaos of everyday life, I've realized that the biggest question is this: Is it worth rushing through life without ever stopping to enjoy it?

I think back to a time when I worked at a bank. Every Friday, without fail, an elderly gentleman, nearly a century old, would arrive to deposit his small check. My coworkers adored him, always asking about his week, nudging him toward conversation. No matter how they framed the question, his answer never changed, never wavered. With a smile, he'd say:

"I'm glad to be above ground!"

That sentence stayed with me. A hundred years on this earth, and his greatest joy was simply being here, existing, seeing another day, living through another moment.
It shifted something in me. How many times do we overlook joy simply because we've decided our circumstances aren't enough? How many times do we let stress, frustration, or boredom steal the beauty of just being alive?

And here's the thing, choosing happiness isn't just about feeling good. It's about survival. When we lean into joy, when we find reasons to laugh, when we lift our own spirits, we heal. Stress eases, health strengthens, life expands into something richer, something lighter.
No matter where we are or what surrounds us, there is joy waiting to be seen. It lives in the laughter we share, in the kindness we extend, in the way we shape the world around us with small, deliberate acts of warmth.

So let's smile, not because life is perfect, but because it is ours. And if we smile first, life has no choice but to smile back.

SHEER CHAI

TREDITIONAL MILK TEA

The tradition of serving tea holds great cultural significance in Uzbekistan. In my upbringing, tea played an essential role in our breakfasts and dinners. Accompanied by vibrant table spreads and a diverse range of food, tea facilitated the consumption of larger meals and provided a sense of comfort. On various occasions, when feeling overly full, the suggestion to drink tea to "push" the food down appeared comical; however, to my surprise, the practice proved effective in creating space for more food.

While growing up in an Arabic-speaking environment for a few years, I frequently heard "shai" being used to refer to tea. In our household, where my dad insisted Farsi was the language of legends, we called it "chai," This was the same name used in those Indian films my parents couldn't get enough of—talk about a cross-cultural tea party! In Farsi, "sheer" means milk, and during special family gatherings, my mother would prepare a beverage called sheer chai; I called it pink chai. It had a delightful pale pink hue with a hint of my favored color, mauve (which may have sparked my affinity for pink). Sheer-chai is a rich, fragrant, sweet milk tea, traditionally topped with a thick cream known as "qaimoak" in Uzbek and Farsi. It is challenging to articulate how indulging in this beverage nourishes the heart and soul, enhancing the enjoyment of family conversations during teatime.

Ingredients

- 4 cups filtered water
- 2 tablespoons organic loose green tea leaves
- ⅛ teaspoon fresh baking soda
- 4-6 ice cubes
- 1 cup pasture-raised organic whole milk
- 2 tablespoons organic raw sugar (adjust to taste)
- ¼ teaspoon freshly ground cardamom
- 2 tablespoons qaimaak or organic whipped heavy cream
- Dried rose petals, for garnish (optional)

Affirmation:

I turn obstacles into momentum. Life doesn't break me, it builds me. Every challenge only proves what I already know: I am limitless.

1. Brew the tea base: In a clean stainless-steel pot, bring 4 cups of water to a gentle boil. Add tea leaves and reduce to a simmer. Let the mixture steep for 25 minutes, stirring every 10 minutes to release the deep flavors.

2. Introduce "The Tea Toss": Once the tea has steeped, add a delicate pinch of baking soda; this is where the transformation begins. Now, practice The Tea Toss: gently scoop the liquid with a ladle, lift it just above the pot, and pour it back in one smooth, confident motion. Repeat this graceful rhythm for about 2 minutes, inviting oxygen and intention into the blend.

Watch closely. As the bubbles begin to blush with a soft pink hue, you've reached the sweet spot, turn off the heat and stir in the ice cubes to calm and set the infusion.

<u>Note:</u> If the bubbles deepen into brown, the base has gone too far..no judgment, just an invitation to begin again. The Tea Toss isn't just technique; it's a dialogue between you and the tea, an embodied reminder that beauty blooms through patience.

3. Infuse the milk: Warm the milk in a separate pot over low heat, being mindful not to scorch it. Add the cooled tea base, then use The Tea Toss method again for 1 minute. The milk will gradually take on a romantic pink tint. Stir in sugar and cardamom, continuing the method for 3 more minutes. Turn off heat.

4. Serve with intention: Ladle the sheer chai into elegant cups. Top each with a spoonful of qaimaak and, if you wish, a gentle scattering of rose petals. Close your eyes, inhale the fragrant steam, and sip slowly, with reverence for the moment.

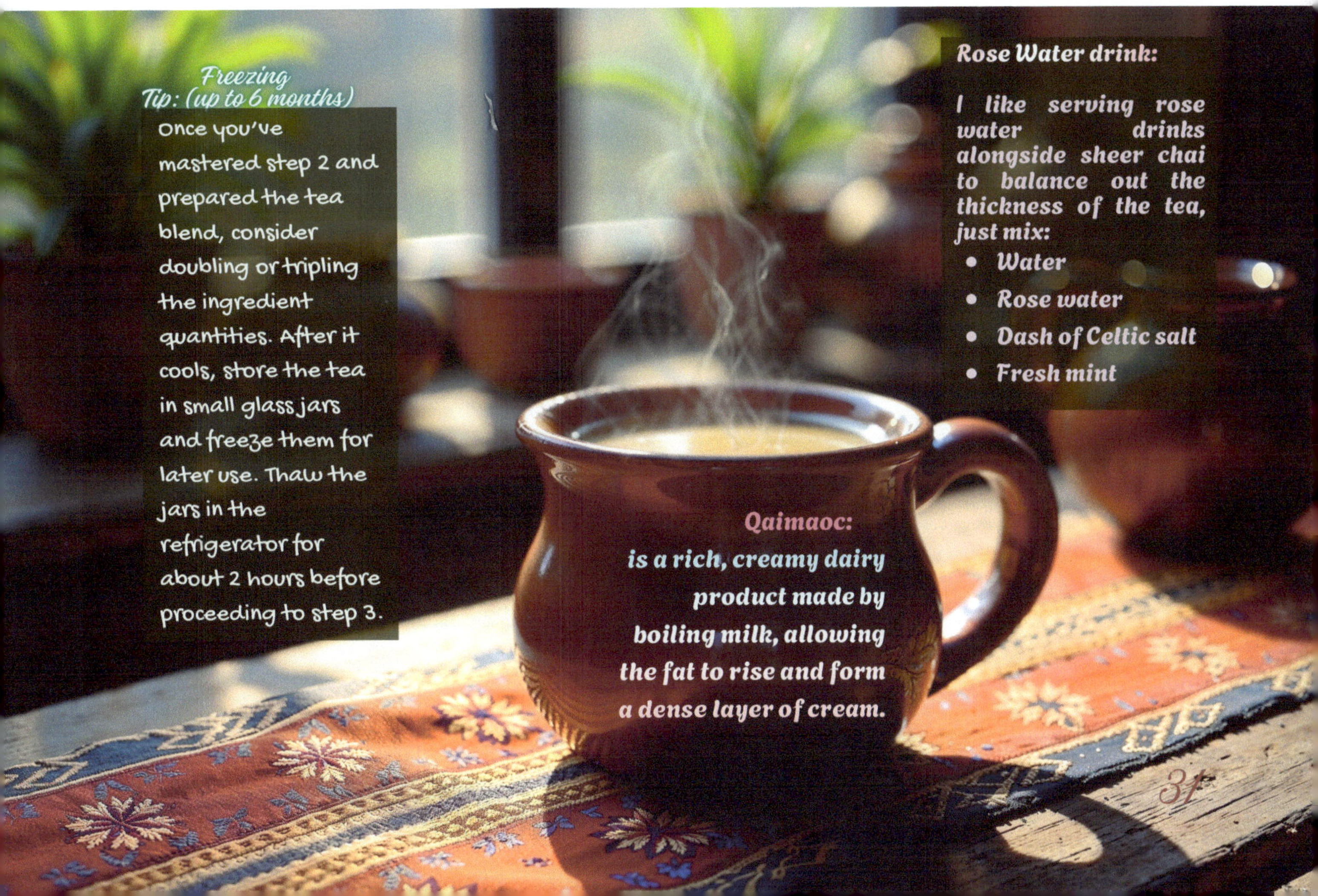

Freezing Tip: (up to 6 months)

Once you've mastered step 2 and prepared the tea blend, consider doubling or tripling the ingredient quantities. After it cools, store the tea in small glass jars and freeze them for later use. Thaw the jars in the refrigerator for about 2 hours before proceeding to step 3.

Rose Water drink:

I like serving rose water drinks alongside sheer chai to balance out the thickness of the tea, just mix:

- Water
- Rose water
- Dash of Celtic salt
- Fresh mint

Qaimaoc:

is a rich, creamy dairy product made by boiling milk, allowing the fat to rise and form a dense layer of cream.

Chill out and cut time: this hack is ice-cold genius!

If there's one thing that keeps my kitchen running, it's this base: onions, carrots, celery, and tomatoes. Prepping it every day? No thanks. So once a month, I make a big batch, freeze it in portions, and suddenly, cooking feels like a breeze.

Now, let's talk about my liver. I like to keep things fresh because, well, that hardworking organ has enough to do without dealing with the effects of long-frozen food. Freezing is fantastic, but beyond six weeks, oxidation kicks in, changing the food's composition and adding extra work for my body. So why not make life easier for this underrated multitasker? Here's how I make it:

1. Caramelize sliced onions until they're deep golden and full of flavor.
2. Add finely chopped carrots and celery, cooking them for a few minutes to soften.
3. Stir in diced tomatoes, a pinch of salt, and some tomato paste for extra richness.
4. Simmer for 5–10 minutes, then let it cool.
5. Freeze in portions so I'm always ready to add a burst of flavor to any meal.

Now, here's a thought, have you ever looked at a simple ingredient and seen its hidden potential? This base, mixed with water, spices, and noodles, can transform into an easy, nourishing soup. But what if we pushed it further? Could a splash of coconut milk take it somewhere unexpected? Could a handful of herbs give it a whole new personality?

Food is more than sustenance, it's creativity, care, and a little bit of adventure. So what's the next way you'll surprise yourself in the kitchen?

Kulchai Namaki, fondly called "salty cookie," is more than a simple biscuit. It holds the essence of tradition, the warmth of nostalgia, and the quiet language of love. When paired with sheer chai, its crisp flakiness and gentle saltiness contrast beautifully with the tea's soothing sweetness, a combination that lingers not just on the palate but in the heart.

For me, Namaki became a bridge; a way to reach across the miles that separated me from my grandfather. He was a man of unwavering values, raised in tradition yet always encouraging of my dreams. Though he visited infrequently, every reunion was precious, and I longed for a way to show him how much he meant to me.

With limited culinary skills, baking Namaki became my love language. Each batch was a silent offering, my hands carefully crafting biscuits that would carry my admiration and gratitude. The moment he tasted them, his smile, genuine and full of appreciation, made every effort worthwhile. It was an unspoken promise woven into layers of golden, flaky dough.

Though he is no longer here, Namaki remains, a testament to our bond, a memory preserved in the aroma of baked biscuits and the comfort of shared moments. It reminds me that love transcends time and distance, living on in the traditions we create and the stories we carry.

Even now, in quiet moments, I imagine setting a cup of sheer chai beside a plate of Namaki, as if he were still here to enjoy them. And in some way, maybe he is—his presence lingering in every crumb, every sip, every memory.

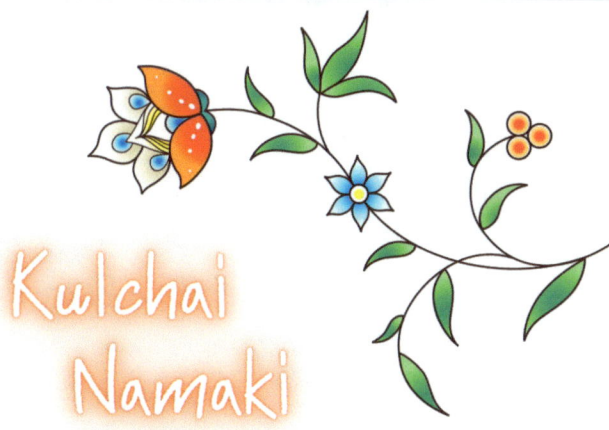

Kulchai Namaki

Growing up in a culturally rich household, I was deeply influenced by my Uzbek parents, who had spent a significant part of their youth in Afghanistan, navigating the complexities of life under challenging circumstances. They brought with them a treasure of traditions, especially revolving around food, which played a central role in our family's life. One of the standout dishes that graced our table was Namaki, a savory bread that embodies the flavors and warmth of Afghan cuisine. The preparation of such meals was not just about nourishment; it was a way for my parents to connect us to their heritage and share the stories of their past.

From my experiences, I've come to realize that facing and overcoming adversity can serve as a catalyst for forging deep, meaningful relationships within a new community. The challenges we faced often opened doors to compassion, understanding, and support from others who had their own stories of resilience. I believe that maintaining a positive outlook in tough times is crucial—not just for personal well-being, but for fostering hope and unity in the face of hardships. In a world full of uncertainty, holding onto hope can illuminate pathways for healing and connection, allowing us to thrive together despite our struggles.

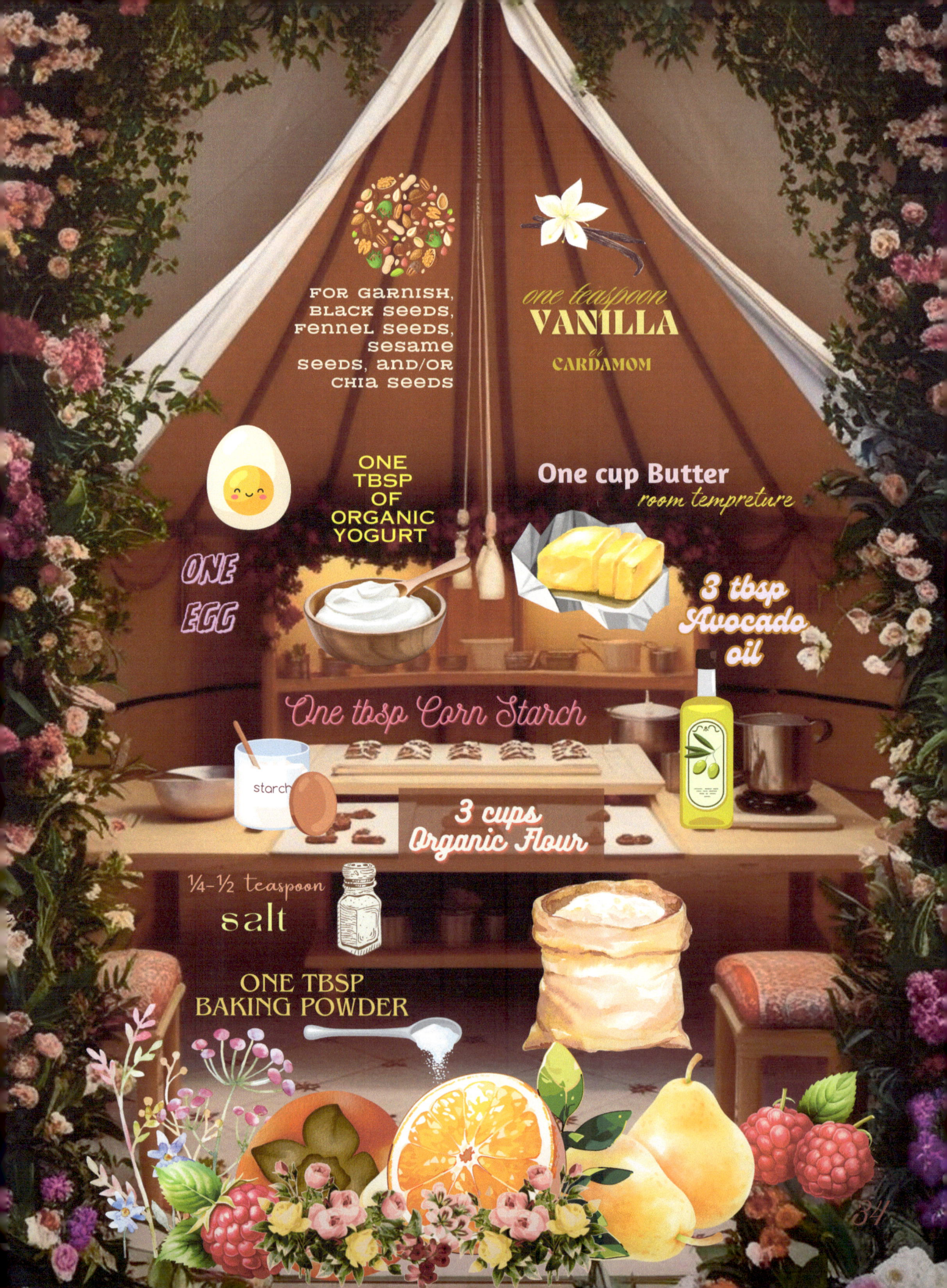

FOR GARNISH, BLACK SEEDS, FENNEL SEEDS, SESAME SEEDS, AND/OR CHIA SEEDS

one teaspoon **VANILLA** *or* **CARDAMOM**

ONE TBSP OF ORGANIC YOGURT

One cup Butter *room tempreture*

ONE EGG

3 tbsp Avocado oil

One tbsp Corn Starch

starch

3 cups Organic Flour

¼–½ teaspoon salt

ONE TBSP BAKING POWDER

34

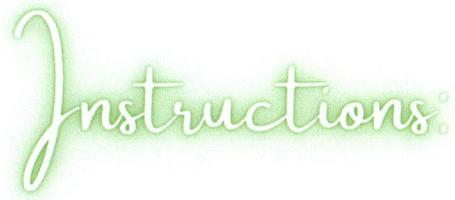

Instructions:

1- Combine butter, avocado oil, egg, and vanilla in a stand mixer or using a hand mixer. Beat the mixture until it becomes light and fluffy. Then, add yogurt and mix for 15 seconds.

2- Mix all the dry ingredients together in a large bowl. Gradually add one cup at a time of the dry mixture to the batter, using a spatula or the paddle attachment if you're using a stand mixer. Mix until the dough is smooth and not sticky.

3- Preheat oven to 350F and line 2 baking pans with baking sheets.

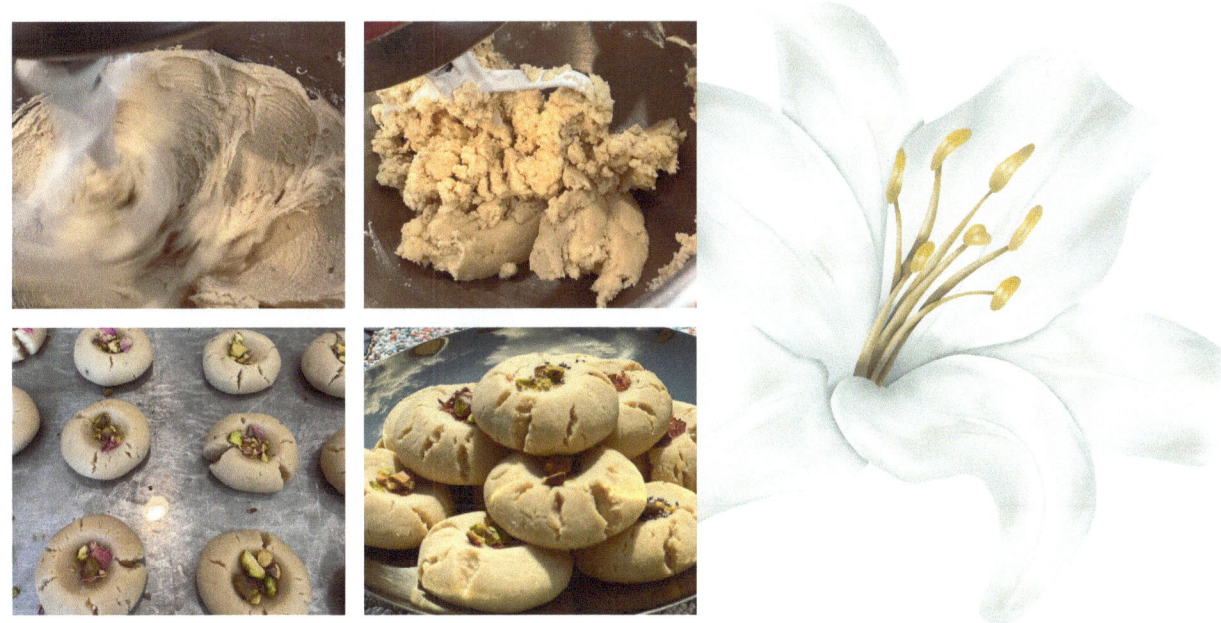

4- For cookie preparation, portion the dough using an ice cream scooper and shape it into balls. Place the balls on a baking pan, then use your thumb to create a dent in the middle and gently flatten them. Next, sprinkle the cookies with seeds and bake at 350°F for 25 minutes. Afterwards, transfer the pans to the top shelf of the oven, raise the temperature to 400°F, and allow the cookies to brown for an additional 2 minutes.

5- Once these treats are removed from the oven, allow them to cool thoroughly and enjoy!

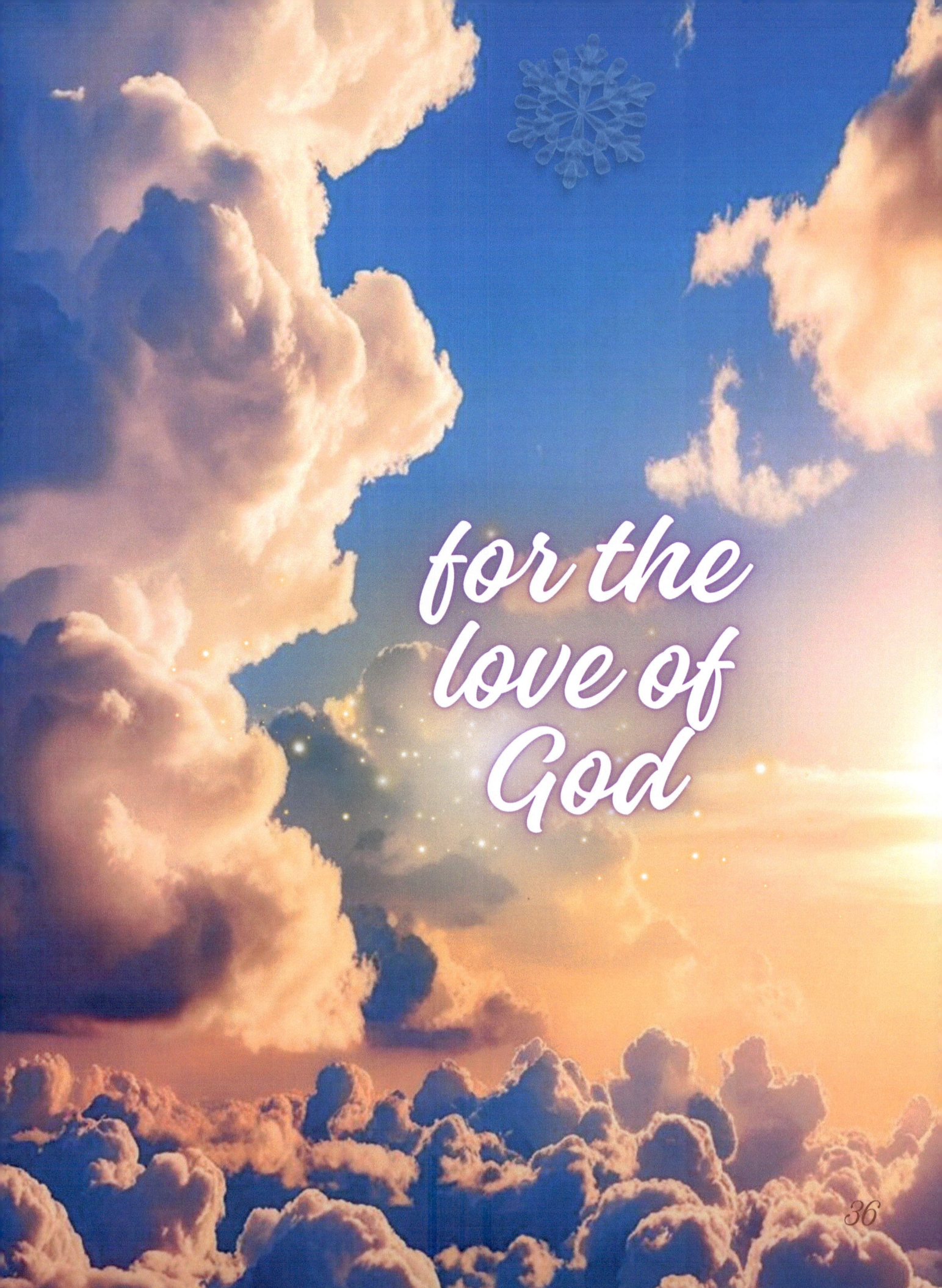

for the
love of
God

As someone who has always detested the idea of limits, restrictions, and rules, I often find myself navigating life in a way that respects the flow of time and the space of others. Just as a traffic light serves as a crucial mechanism for ensuring safety on the roads, I discover a sense of security within the boundaries of my beliefs. Surrendering to a higher power and acknowledging a force greater than myself remarkably alleviates the weight of responsibility that often feels overwhelming.

From my perspective, I am composed of both a physical body and a deeper, spiritual essence. Focusing solely on my physical being can lead to an unfulfilled existence and a lack of true happiness. My spirit craves companionship and nurturing beyond the material realm. Daily practices such as prayer and reflection provide a vital cleansing for my soul, addressing my intrinsic needs as a living creature.

Moreover, embracing and attempting to understand the importance of rules allows me to navigate life with less mental clutter and overthinking. This holistic approach helps me cultivate a balanced existence, one that honors both my physical presence and my spiritual journey. In doing so, I foster a deeper connection with the world around me and with the divine, leading to a more harmonious and fulfilling life.

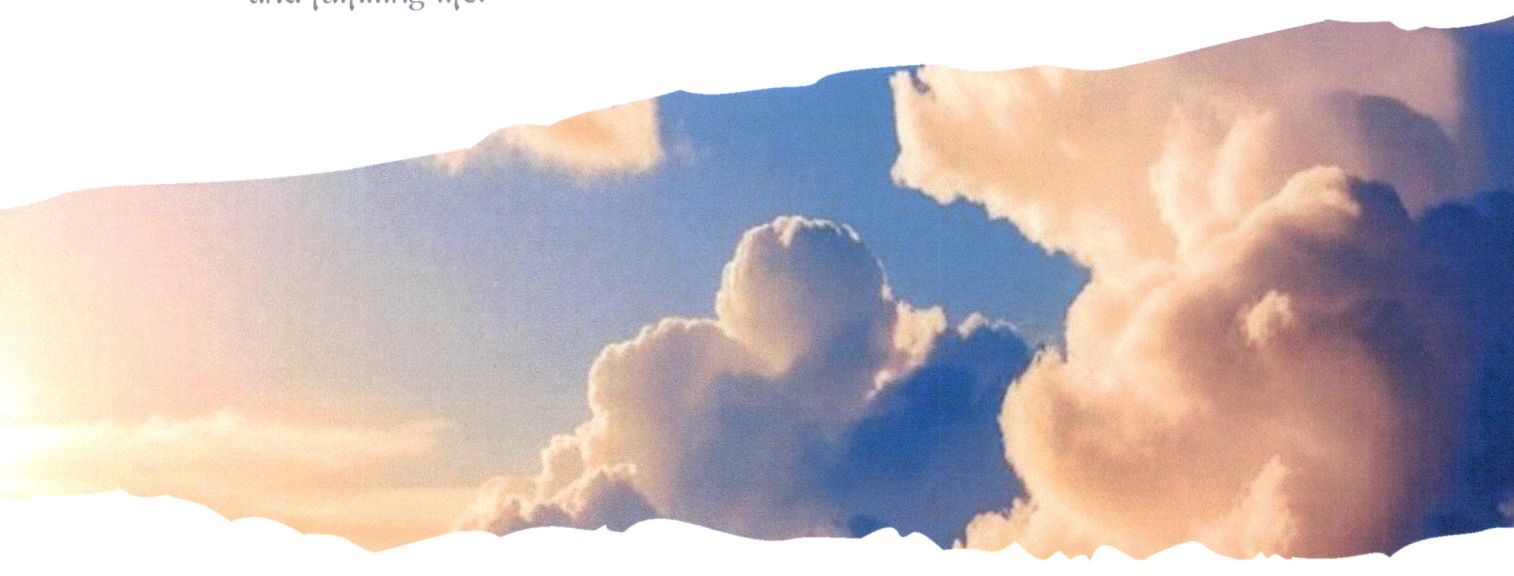

Drama & Diamonds:
The Heat Beneath the Glamour

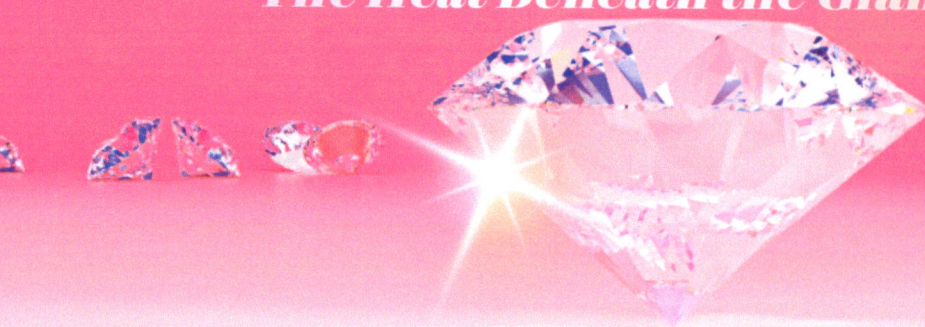
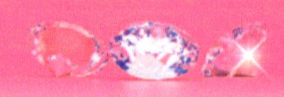

I arrive at family gatherings and friendly get-togethers with nothing but noble intentions, a peaceful envoy on a mission of joy, armed with a sincere smile and the quiet hope of effortless laughter and warm conversation.

But reality, as always, has a taste for theatrics.

Like clockwork, I find myself unwillingly drafted into an unscripted social spectacle, where tension swells faster than I can process it. One moment, I'm reaching for a harmless appetizer; Next, I didn't just step, I stumbled, no, I fell into a scene dense with raised eyebrows and silent judgment, loaded comments, and the kind of atmosphere where even casual banter turns into a battlefield of veiled meanings and strategic silence.

And here's the kicker, I don't even know how it happens. I, the sworn advocate of harmony, seem destined to orbit chaos like a planet caught in an unpredictable gravitational pull. Perhaps I radiate an accidental aura of intrigue. Maybe gatherings are simply designed to ensure no one leaves unscathed. Or maybe *just maybe* this is the price of being interesting.

At first, I told myself these moments were harmless, temporary disruptions, nothing more than an unfortunate coincidence. But as the whispers outlasted the evening, as the conversations stretched beyond the room and morphed into exaggerated retellings, I began to notice the pattern.

These days, it isn't just fleeting gossip behind closed doors; it's digital ink spilling across social media, transforming moments into narratives, reshaping words into controversy, casting me into a story I never asked to be in. And suddenly, weeks later, I find myself stumbling upon versions of me, versions so distorted they feel like strangers.

Somewhere along the way, we stopped meeting to connect and started gathering for spectacle. Laughter was replaced with anticipation, the thrill of who will say what, who will misstep, who will be caught in the tangled web of assumptions and carefully crafted drama. It's no longer about closeness, it's about consumption. And the more we indulge in this cycle, the more we sacrifice the very thing that made human connection beautiful in the first place.

For a long time, I tried to resist it. I tried shrinking away, staying silent, believing that avoidance was the antidote to chaos. But I realize now; running isn't the answer. Redefining the rules is.

So, instead of letting the noise dictate my story, I choose to rewrite it. I refuse to be a passive character in someone else's orchestrated drama. I won't drift in the tides of rumor or let my presence be shaped by whispers. I will stand, unwavering, not as a player, not as a victim, but as the force that rewrites the narrative entirely.

In a world obsessed with spectacle, I choose truth, not carefully curated, but raw. Not in hesitation, but in certainty. Because reality is only a performance if you let it be.

A Culinary Catastrophe:
Rogue Pistachio Reverie
with
Cardamom & Saffron Ice Cream

Inspired by the velvet folds of qatayif, this rogue rendition dares to dream in pistachio. silence.

Surviving the whirlwind of social theatrics and inevitable heartbreak, what better way to reclaim joy than with a dessert that folds softness into rebellion? When life gets messy, the kitchen becomes a sanctuary, a place where frustration simmers into creativity, and chaos transforms into something golden, layered, and quietly victorious.

Time to channel that beautiful madness into pure culinary magic. Imagine a saffron-tinged semolina pancake, thin, golden, and unapologetically tender, soaked in cardamom syrup and folded like a whispered secret. At its heart lies a pistachio cream so lush it feels like velvet defiance. And perched on top? A scoop of cardamom ice cream, cool and fragrant, melting into the folds like forgiveness.

This isn't just dessert, it's a declaration. A plated act of reclamation. A Rogue Pistachio Reverie.

So grab your whisk, embrace the glorious mess, and let's create something unforgettable. With every spoonful of aromatic ice cream and each indulgent bite of saffron-soaked pancake, we'll redefine comfort, proving that the most dazzling flavors arise from life's most chaotic, unfiltered moments.

a Deep Thought

"A wise man never plays the sap-but the real Trick is knowing when to put on the act." ~ Someone who understood the art of the game

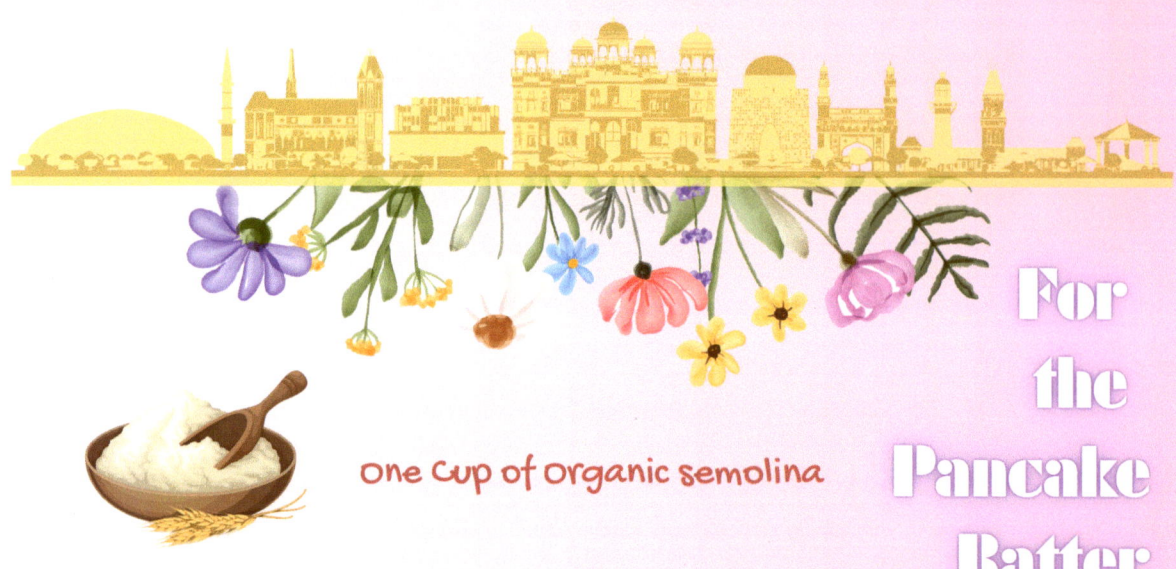

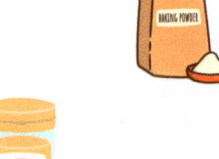 One Cup of Organic semolina

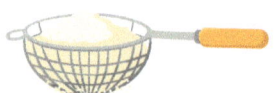 1/2 Cup of organic all-purpose Flour

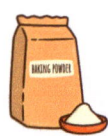 One Teaspoon Baking Powder

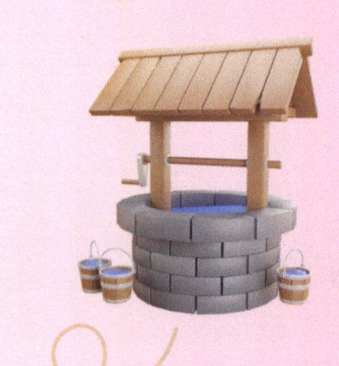

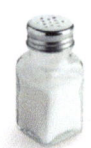 1/2 tsp turmeric powder

pinch of Salt

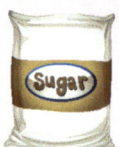 two tbsp Sugar

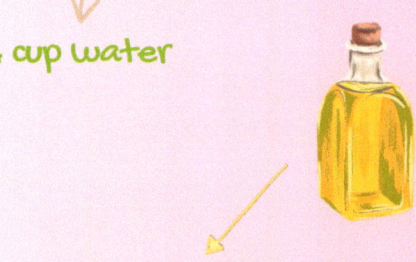 1/4 cup water

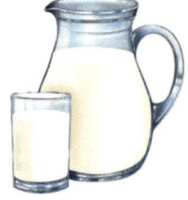 1 1/2 cups milk

1/4 cup neutral oil

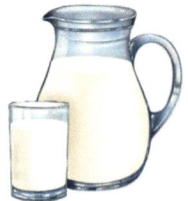 1/2 tsp orange blossom water (optional)

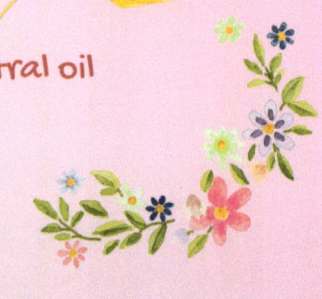

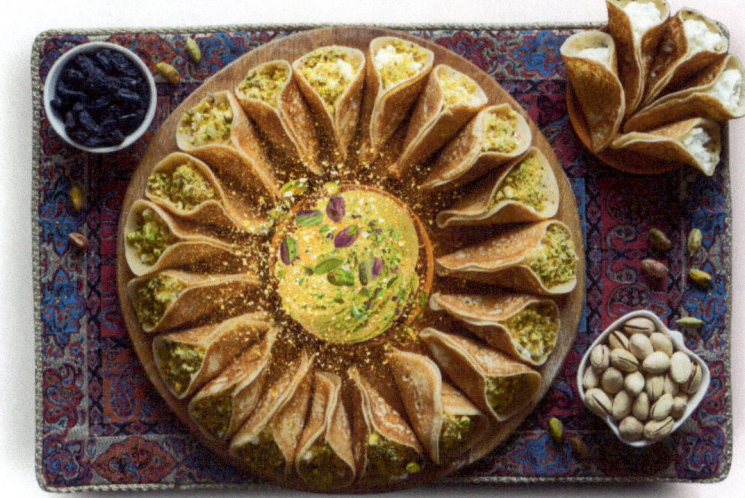

For the Cardamom Syrup

- ½ cup water
- ½ cup sugar
- 4—5 crushed cardamom pods
- 1 tsp rosewater
- Squeeze of lemon juice

For the Pistachio Cream

- ½ cup pistachio paste
- ¼ cup mascarpone or labneh
- 1 tbsp honey or date syrup
- Pinch of salt

For Assembly

- Cardamom and Saffran Ice Cream (Recipe next page)
- Crushed pistachios
- Dried rose petals
- Edible gold dust (optional)

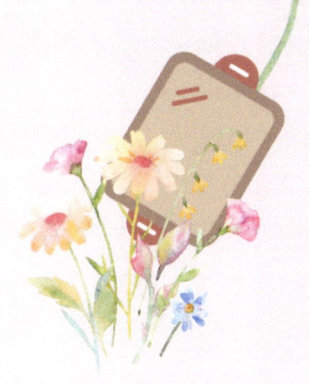

Instructions:

1. Make the Batter
 Whisk semolina, flour, turmeric, baking powder, salt, and sugar. Add milk, water, orange blossom, and oil. Mix until smooth. Let rest 15—20 minutes.

2. Cook the Pancakes
 Heat a nonstick pan over medium-low. Pour a thin layer of batter, swirl to spread. Cook until golden and set. Don't flip. Repeat and keep warm.

3. Prepare the Syrup
 Simmer water, sugar, and cardamom until slightly thickened. Add rosewater and lemon juice. Let cool.

4. Make the Pistachio Cream
 Blend pistachio paste, mascarpone, honey, and salt until smooth. Chill.

5. Assemble
Brush each pancake with warm syrup. Spread pistachio cream. Fold gently.
Top with ice cream, crushed pistachios, rose petals, and gold dust.
Take a moment to appreciate the beauty of your dessert; a visual feast that promises to elevate your spirits and shift your mood from any mishap to a feeling of delight, ready to embrace the next party drama!

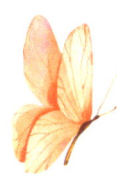

As someone who draws inspiration from the vast diversity of cultures and experiences the world has to offer, I find great joy in creating my own unique stuff. However, there are two areas where I have yet to achieve mastery: crafting flower arrangements and making homemade ice cream.

To streamline the process and ensure top-notch quality, I've decided to opt for a premium, full-fat organic vanilla ice cream as my base. This recipe is a game changer—its rich, creamy texture and vibrant flavors are simply unparalleled. Trust me; it's a creamy madness that will truly rock your world!

Cardamom & Saffran Ice Cream:

Ingredients:

- One pint of vanilla ice cream
- ½ a cup of heavy cream
- Two tablespoons of condensed milk
- One tablespoon of freshly ground cardamom
- One pinch of saffron (crushed with fingers)
- ¼ cup of roughly ground pistachios

Instructions:

1. In a stand mixer fitted with a paddle attachment or a large-capacity food processor, combine the ice cream, heavy cream, and condensed milk.

2. Mix the ingredients on a low to medium speed, allowing them to blend thoroughly. The goal here is to achieve a creamy consistency that's almost like soft-serve ice cream.

3. Once the mixture reaches the desired consistency, carefully add the remaining ingredients. Take a moment to ensure everything is evenly distributed before mixing.

4. For the next step, mix the ingredients gently yet thoroughly. If you are using the stand mixer, mix for about 10 seconds, infusing some extra love into this process. If you opt for the food processor, pulse it only three times.

5. After mixing, transfer this luscious mixture into a larger bowl, and finally, it's time to start crafting this creamy creation!

Faithful From This Side of The Page

We live in an age where loyalty has been rebranded as self-interest.

People say they're loyal, but what they mean is: *I'll stay as long as it serves me.*

Love has become a mirror, reflecting only what we want to see.

And truth? It bends to comfort.

Picture a single sheet of paper. On one side, it reads a 6. Flip it, and it becomes a 9. Two people, standing on opposite ends, see the same symbol differently. That's perspective. But what cuts deeper is when someone who knows your story, your scars, your silence, starts arguing from the other side. Not because they're confused. But because they've chosen to stand with the opposition. They look at your 6 and say, "No, it's a 9." Not out of misunderstanding, but out of convenience.

That's not disagreement. That's disloyalty.

True loyalty means *I love you more than I love being right.*

It means *I'll hold your truth even when it's inconvenient.*

But today, loyalty often comes with fine print: *I'm with you... until it costs me comfort, reputation, or control.*

And that's where the rooftop story comes in.

In Afghanistan, on a warm, clear night, a family sleeps on the rooftop—tradition, stars, silence. The mother lies in the center. On her left: her son and his wife. On her right: her daughter and son-in-law. She turns to her daughter-in-law and says, "Move away from my son-you're making him hot." Then turns to her daughter and says, "Hold your husband-it's cold."

Same rooftop. Same night. But the rules? Written with one heart. Her son's comfort matters. Her daughter's warmth matters. But the daughter-in-law's presence? A problem. Not because of temperature. But her feelings don't factor into the mother-in-law's emotional economy. Her love doesn't extend outward; it loops back to herself.

The daughter-in-law, quiet but sharp, whispers:

"May the heavens witness, one rooftop, two winds. One heart embraced, another erased."

It wasn't about sides. It was about selective love.

It was about how some people only extend care when it reflects well on them.

They love you when you're an extension of their comfort.

But the moment your existence requires empathy, they retreat.

And that's the real betrayal.

Not the stranger who disagrees.

But the one who knows your truth and still chooses themselves.

Disloyalty is the friend who demands your loyalty when they are shivering, yet abandons you when the chill is yours. They expect you to stand firm in their storm, but when the same storm finds you, they step to the other side. Same rooftop, same people, yet the wind shifts, and the rules change

Faithfulness doesn't mean perfection.

   It means presence.

   It means *I see you, even when it's easier not to.*

   And in this world of shifting truths and self-serving love,

the ones who stay aren't the ones who agree,

   they're the ones who refuse to flip the page against you.

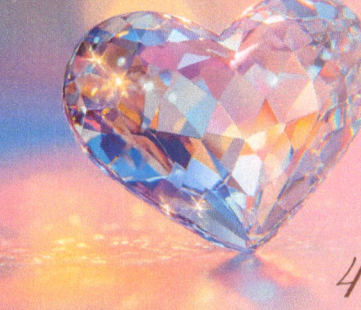

Men of Silent Steel

They walk like the ground owes them nothing. Shoulders squared, eyes steady, hands that know the weight of things, tools, grief, a child asleep in the backseat. You notice them not because they speak, but because the room adjusts when they enter. There's a kind of masculine stillness that doesn't ask for attention; it earns it.

I grew up watching men like that. My father, my brothers—men who didn't flinch when the world leaned hard. Later, I'd see echoes of them in the man who shares my table, and in the boy who's learning how to lace his shoes with quiet pride. They didn't talk about pain. They didn't name exhaustion. They carried it like a second skin, stitched into their posture, folded into their silence. I learned early that strength wasn't loud. It was the way they stayed.

But staying came at a cost. I saw it in the skipped meals, the unopened vitamins, the cough that lingered too long. I saw it in the way they'd drive everyone else to the doctor but never schedule their own check-up. I saw it in the quiet rituals of self-neglect-work first, rest later, care never.

And still, they were beautiful. Not in the way magazines pretend to understand, but in the way a man becomes a landscape-weathered, useful, enduring. You could build a life around them. You could fall asleep knowing they'd still be there in the morning.

But I also knew this: even the strongest beams crack if no one checks for termites. Even the most loyal men need tending. Not because they're weak, but because they're human. And somewhere along the way, someone taught them that being cared for made them less.

It doesn't.

There's nothing more magnetic than a man who lets himself be kept. Who learns the language of rest. Who lets love land without suspicion. Who understands that wellness isn't a luxury-it's part of the legacy he's building.

So I cook. I ask twice. I leave things on the counter that say, "I see you." I don't wait for him to ask. I don't need him to explain. I just make it easy for him to stay whole.

Because the men who hold everything deserve to be held. And the silence they carry deserves to be answered—not with noise, but with care that knows how to listen.

SLEEP

We wake up, dive in, and before we know it, we're moving fast. The coffee kicks in, the emails pile up, and the to-do list grows legs. It's modern life: efficient, relentless, a blur of dopamine hits and calendar reminders. We've gotten so good at productivity, we've nearly forgotten how to pause.

But the body? The body hasn't forgotten. It keeps score, gently at first: that afternoon slump, the extra sugar craving, the sudden loss of sparkle in our eyes. These tiny signals are less about laziness and more like love letters from our nervous system, whispering: rest me.

And still, we scroll. We binge. We stare into blue light, disconnected from the natural rhythm that once cradled us, the moonrise, the hush of twilight, the stars that used to remind us: it's time.

Sleep isn't weakness or indulgence. It's ceremony. It's chemistry. It's the backstage crew restoring every cell, sweeping up after the madness of the day. It balances hormones, repairs tissue, regulates weight, and sharpens the mind. Lack of it? It's not just about feeling groggy-it can dim your mood, strain your heart, and invite imbalance into places you didn't expect.

But when we honor sleep, when we dim the lights, silence the buzz, and let go, something magical happens. Focus returns. Mood lifts. The immune system resets. The body hums in tune again.

So tonight, reclaim the ritual. Let the lights glow lower. Let the noise fade. Step outside if you can. Let your eyes meet a star or two. Let them pull your thoughts into stillness. Then climb into the quiet, tuck yourself in—not just to bed, but back into rhythm.

Sleep isn't just where the day ends! it's where you begin again.

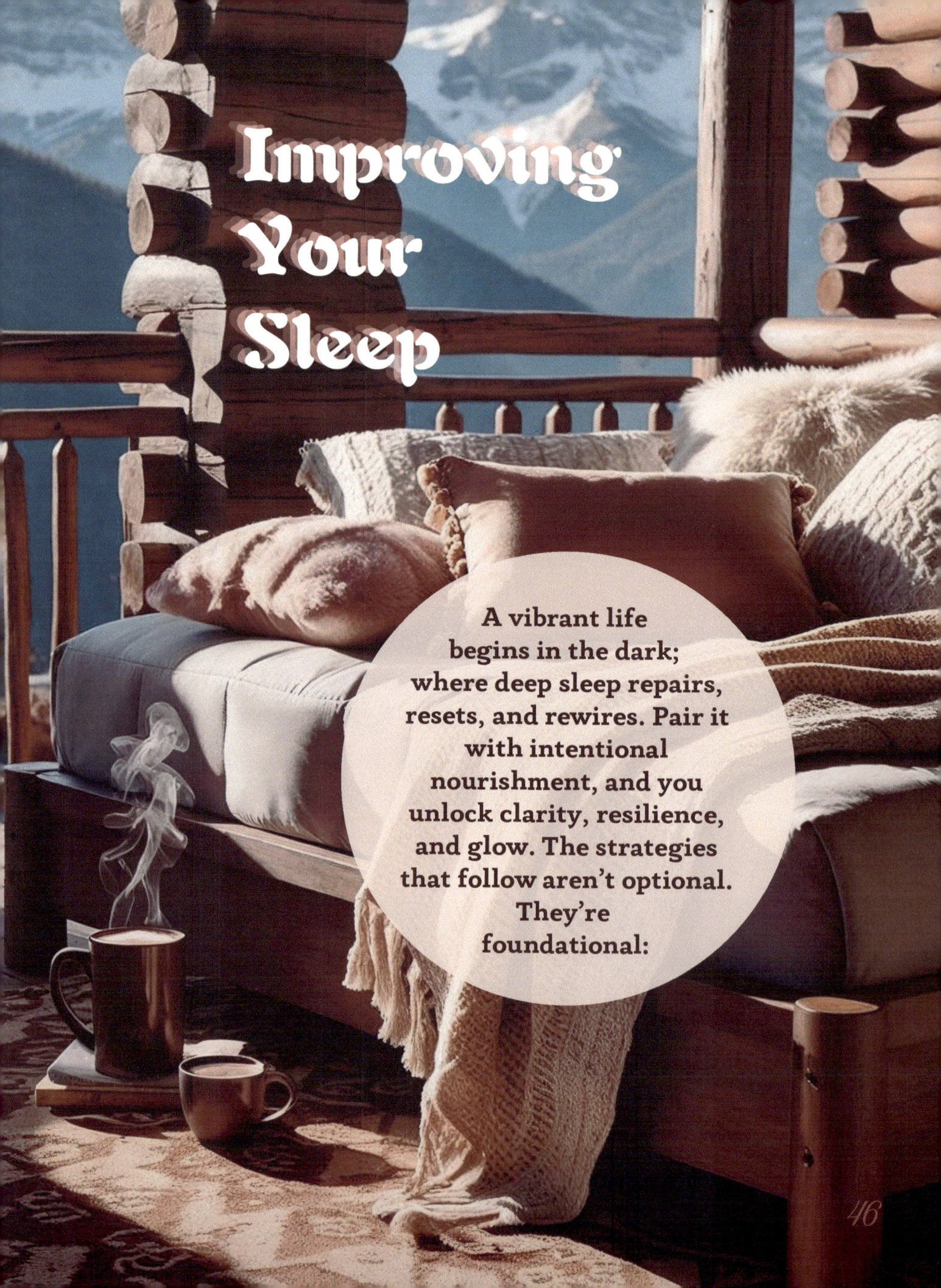

Improving Your Sleep

A vibrant life begins in the dark; where deep sleep repairs, resets, and rewires. Pair it with intentional nourishment, and you unlock clarity, resilience, and glow. The strategies that follow aren't optional. They're foundational:

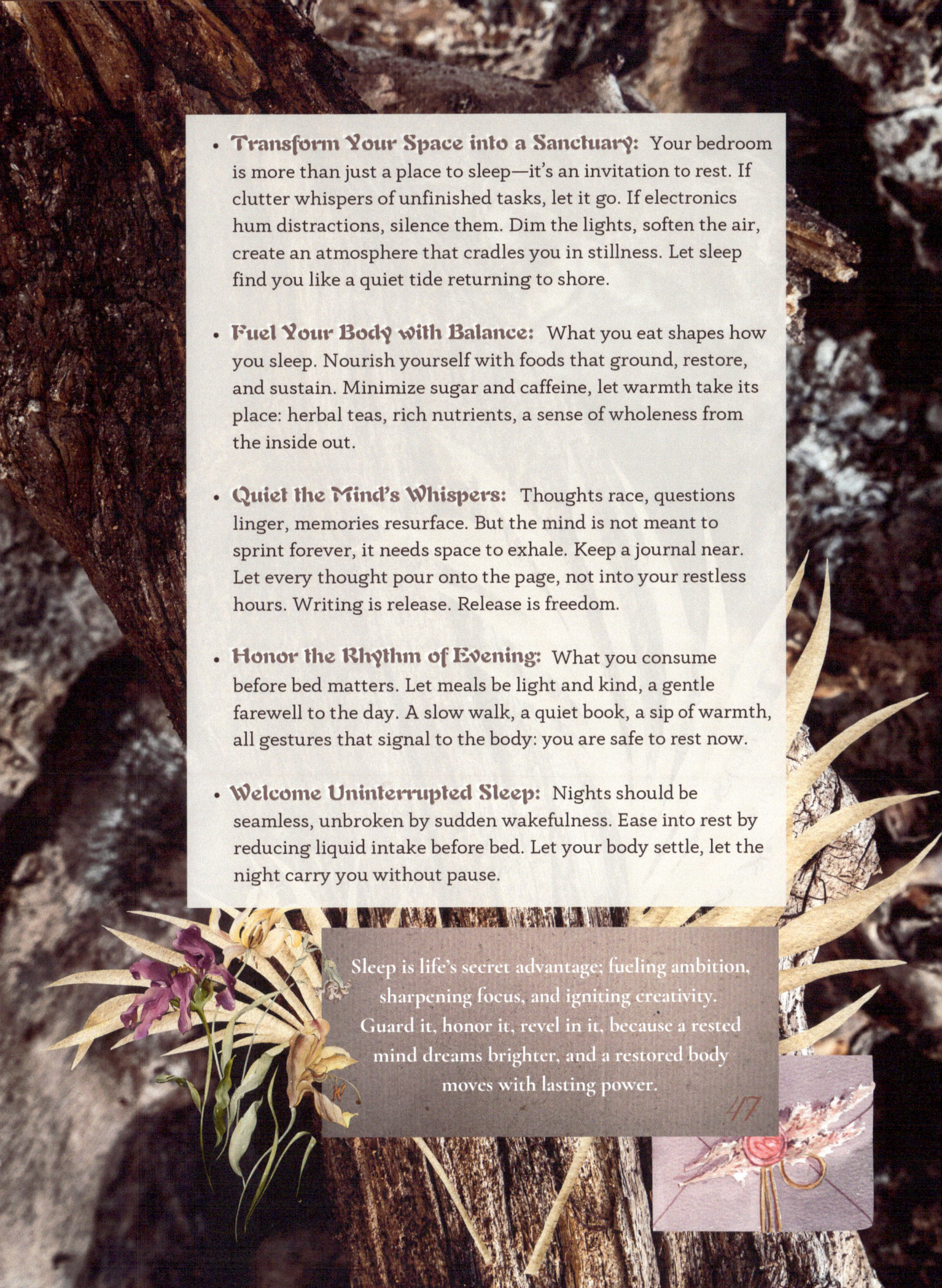

- **Transform Your Space into a Sanctuary:** Your bedroom is more than just a place to sleep—it's an invitation to rest. If clutter whispers of unfinished tasks, let it go. If electronics hum distractions, silence them. Dim the lights, soften the air, create an atmosphere that cradles you in stillness. Let sleep find you like a quiet tide returning to shore.

- **Fuel Your Body with Balance:** What you eat shapes how you sleep. Nourish yourself with foods that ground, restore, and sustain. Minimize sugar and caffeine, let warmth take its place: herbal teas, rich nutrients, a sense of wholeness from the inside out.

- **Quiet the Mind's Whispers:** Thoughts race, questions linger, memories resurface. But the mind is not meant to sprint forever, it needs space to exhale. Keep a journal near. Let every thought pour onto the page, not into your restless hours. Writing is release. Release is freedom.

- **Honor the Rhythm of Evening:** What you consume before bed matters. Let meals be light and kind, a gentle farewell to the day. A slow walk, a quiet book, a sip of warmth, all gestures that signal to the body: you are safe to rest now.

- **Welcome Uninterrupted Sleep:** Nights should be seamless, unbroken by sudden wakefulness. Ease into rest by reducing liquid intake before bed. Let your body settle, let the night carry you without pause.

Sleep is life's secret advantage: fueling ambition, sharpening focus, and igniting creativity. Guard it, honor it, revel in it, because a rested mind dreams brighter, and a restored body moves with lasting power.

47

The Night Doesn't Knock

It just slips in.

While you're still scrolling.

While your mind is arguing with itself about tomorrow.

While your body, loyal, tired, waits for permission to shut down.

You don't even notice the shift at first. Maybe a longer blink. A sigh. The sudden weight of your limbs. Something inside you whispers, Enough. And whether you listen or not, night begins its quiet takeover.

And that's when sleep finds you. Not like a guest, more like a secret. It tiptoes in, rearranging the furniture of your body in the dark, fine-tuning things you didn't even know were off. Memories. Mood. Strength. Balance.

It doesn't ask your permission. It restores you anyway.

One lesson in particular has clung to me since middle school. My teacher, sharp, no-nonsense, warned us against cramming before an exam. "Study before bed," she said. "Your brain will do the rest while you sleep."

Back then, I wasn't sure whether to believe her. But I tried. And something clicked. The next morning, answers felt like they were waiting for me. My thoughts had been ironed smooth, crisp at the edges, as if some unseen librarian had stayed up all night filing every idea into the perfect place.

That was the first time I realized sleep wasn't just rest. It was strategy. Power. Alignment. A quiet partner in every version of success I'd ever want.

And even now, after long days and wild seasons, I still marvel at its mystery. Sleep is where we vanish, then return better. It's the unspoken agreement between body and soul: You take care of me, I'll take care of you.

So tonight, let the day fall away. Let the stars take over the storytelling. Let sleep do its silent, extraordinary work.

Tomorrow is waiting, but you don't have to chase it.

Close your eyes, and let it come to you.

The benefits of sleep extend far beyond memory retention. When restful nights are prioritized, overall energy levels are increased. Additionally, sleep strengthens the immune system is stronger, elevates mental clarity, and nurtures creativity, allowing one to approach challenges with fresh perspectives and innovative solutions.

Continue:

Getting enough sleep significantly boosts emotional well-being, helping to reduce feelings of anxiety and irritability that can often affect one's mood. This transformation leads to a happier and healthier version of oneself, encouraging a greater appreciation for self-care as an essential part of life. Additionally, making sleep a priority has a delightful side effect, it increases libido and enriches the overall enjoyment of intimate experiences.

One significant lifestyle change that I both celebrate and struggle with is reducing my coffee intake. Although I once relied on caffeine to get through the day, this adjustment has had a remarkable impact on my sleep quality. I now sleep more soundly, experiencing deeper rest that rejuvenates my body and mind. By prioritizing sleep in my life, I feel as though I have unlocked the door to better health, liberating myself from the burdens of weight gain and chronic diseases.

Inadequate sleep not only affects physical health but also impairs cognitive function, leading to difficulties in processing information, making sound decisions, and regulating emotions. Acknowledging the significance of sleep has been a pivotal moment in my journey toward overall wellness, motivating me to cultivate restorative practices that empower me to live life to the fullest.

PLANNING *TUESDAY*

- Grow your own seed sprouts: Choose alfalfa, mung bean, or radish seeds. Rinse, soak for 6-8 hours, and then place them in a sprouting jar. Rinse and drain twice daily, and in a few days, enjoy fresh sprouts in salads or sandwiches.

- Bake a loaf of homemade bread, choosing your preferred recipe.

- Find a pancake mix recipe and prepare the dry ingredients to have on hand for the week.

- Plan next Tuesday's menu, ensuring a balanced breakfast, lunch, and dinner for everyone's preferences.

Affirmation:

I embrace my unique beauty, celebrating every aspect of myself that makes me who I am.

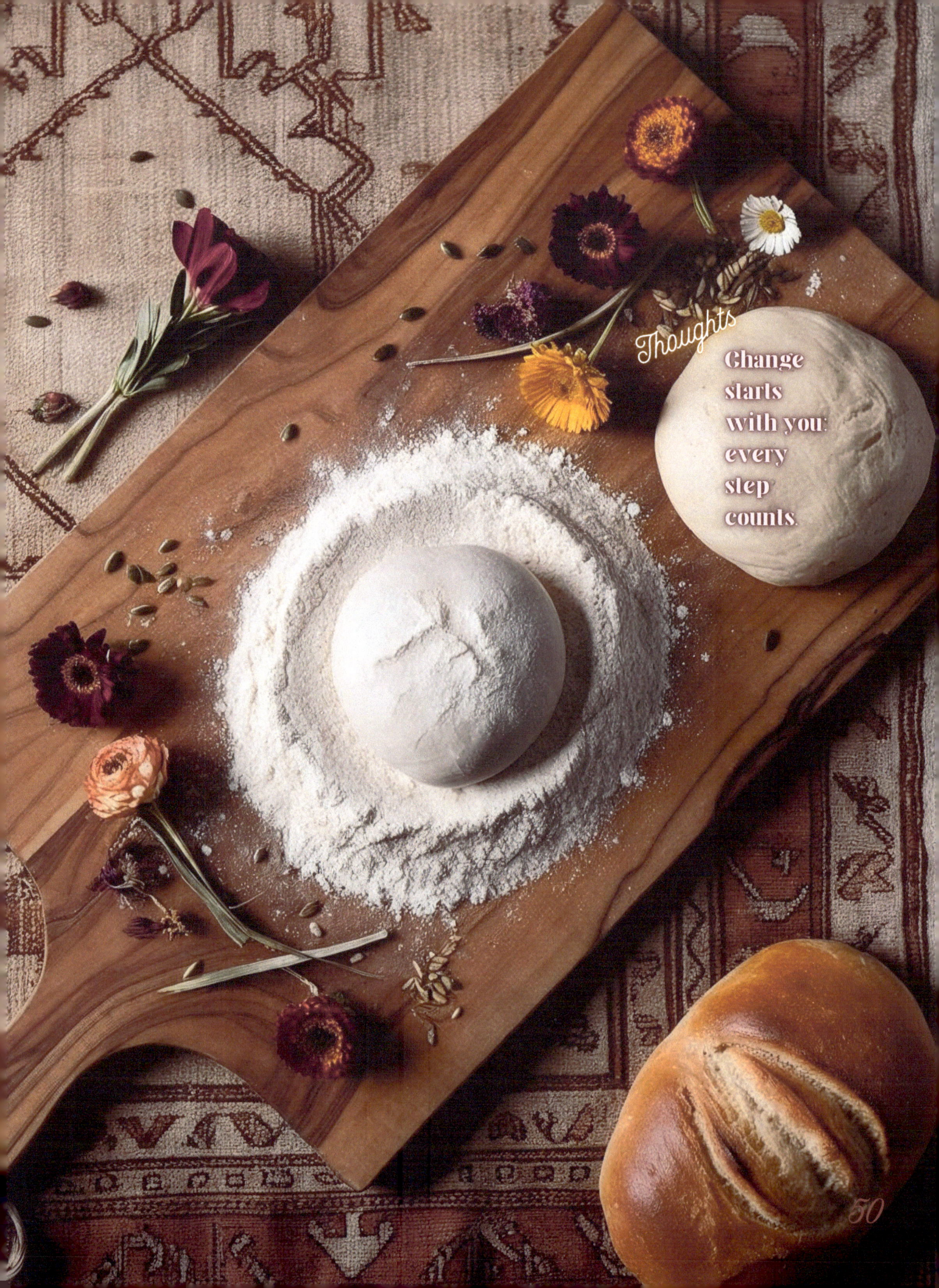

Thoughts

**Change
starts
with you:
every
step
counts.**

50

Uzbek Na'an

The magical
whiff of freshly baked bread! It's
like a time-travel ticket straight to
the golden days of my childhood. Of
all the bread I've had the pleasure
of gobbling down, Uzbek bread is the
MVP in my heart—hands down, one
of the yummiest creations ever to
grace my taste buds!

Growing up, I often heard that every chef adds their
unique touch to their cooking, which seems to be an art
form in its own right. Unfortunately, my attempts to
recreate traditional Uzbek bread never quite captured
that magic. While it would turn out beautifully fluffy
and flavorful on the day of baking, it seemed to fall
victim to time, becoming chewy and tough (and not in a
desirable way) by the next day.

In my quest for perfection, I experimented with various
ingredients. I tried adding eggs and milk to enrich the
dough, but instead of achieving the desired bread
texture, I ended up with a cake-like consistency, which
was not what I envisioned.

But giving up was never on the menu! One fine day, my eyes
landed on a dreamy, creamy ingredient chilling in the fridge,
and I thought, "It's go time!" The outcome? Bread that's as
fluffy as a cloud on a summer day, yet sturdy enough to
whisper, "I'm in it for the long haul." The best part? This
bread stays scrumptiously delightful for 2 to 3 days post-
baking. Each nibble delivers a warm hug of tradition,
whisking me away to the heart of Uzbek cuisine and leaving
a lingering sense of joy that lasts way beyond the first bite.

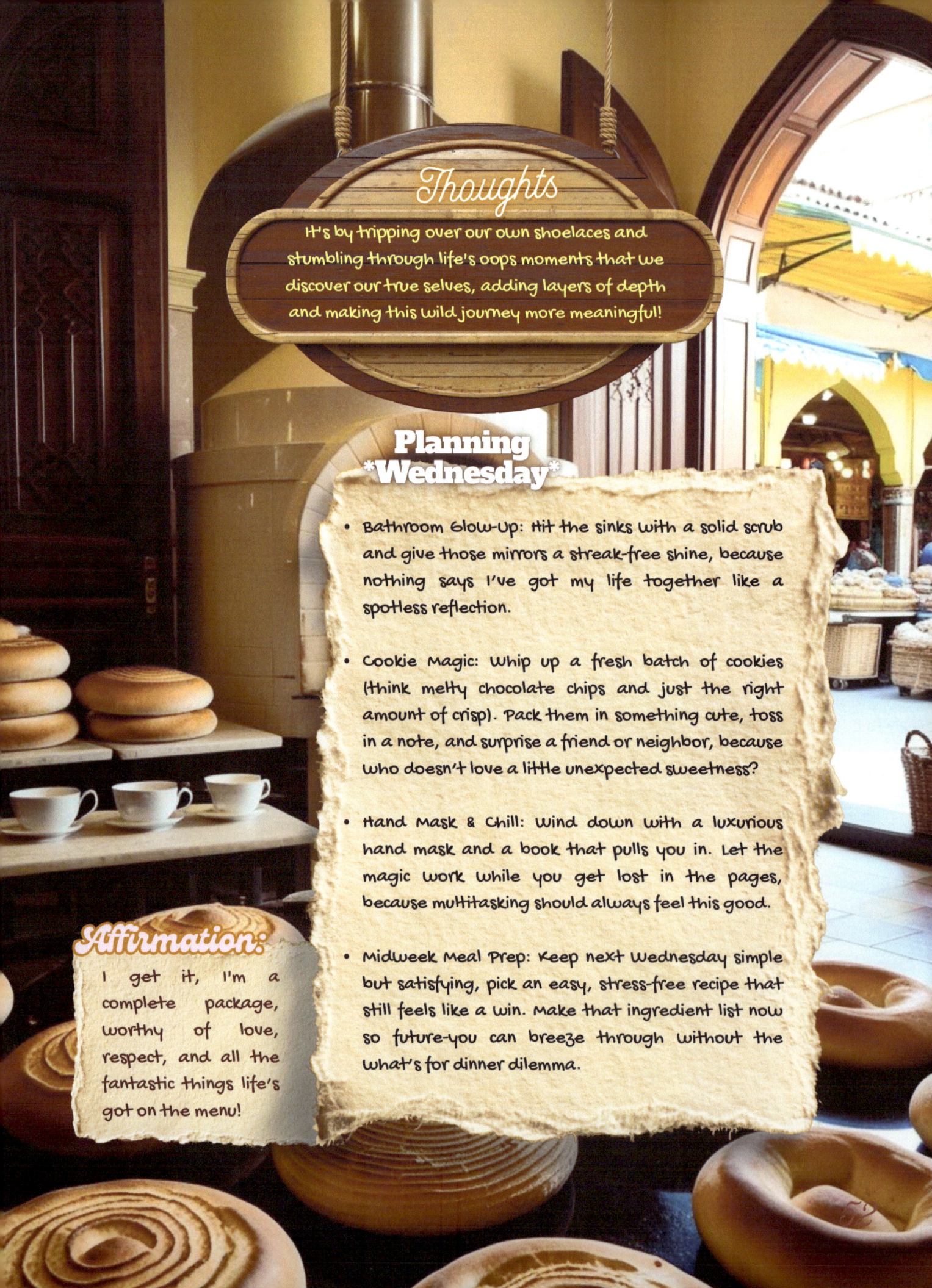

Thoughts

It's by tripping over our own shoelaces and stumbling through life's oops moments that we discover our true selves, adding layers of depth and making this wild journey more meaningful!

Planning
Wednesday

- **Bathroom Glow-Up:** Hit the sinks with a solid scrub and give those mirrors a streak-free shine, because nothing says I've got my life together like a spotless reflection.

- **Cookie Magic:** Whip up a fresh batch of cookies (think melty chocolate chips and just the right amount of crisp). Pack them in something cute, toss in a note, and surprise a friend or neighbor, because who doesn't love a little unexpected sweetness?

- **Hand Mask & Chill:** Wind down with a luxurious hand mask and a book that pulls you in. Let the magic work while you get lost in the pages, because multitasking should always feel this good.

- **Midweek Meal Prep:** Keep next Wednesday simple but satisfying, pick an easy, stress-free recipe that still feels like a win. Make that ingredient list now so future-you can breeze through without the what's for dinner dilemma.

Affirmation:

I get it, I'm a complete package, worthy of love, respect, and all the fantastic things life's got on the menu!

Ingredients:

16 OZ LUKEWARM WATER

ONE TABLESPOON ORGANIC RAW SUGAR

TWO TEASPOONS ACTIVE YEAST

5-6 CUPS ORGANIC UNBLEACHED BREAD FLOUR (OR ALL-PURPOSE FLOUR) SOME EXTRA FOR DUSTING

BLACK SEEDS, CHIA SEEDS, OR SESAME SEEDS

TWO TEASPOONS OF SALT

THREE TABLESPOONS ORGANIC MAYONNAISE

(the dreamy creamy ingredient)

ONE ORGANIC PASTURE-RAISED EGG

FIVE TABLESPOONS MELTED BUTTER

1. Prepare the Yeast Mixture: Start by pouring warm water into the bowl of a stand mixer fitted with the paddle attachment, or into a large mixing bowl if you're mixing by hand. Add sugar and active dry yeast to the water. Optionally, this is a great moment to take a moment of reflection or say a little prayer for good results. Stir gently to dissolve the sugar and yeast, then allow the mixture to rest for about 10 minutes. During this time, you should begin to see bubbles and foam forming on the surface, which indicates that the yeast is activated (If the yeast doesn't produce bubbles, it may indicate that it is no longer active.)

2. Combine the Ingredients: Once the yeast mixture is bubbly, add 2 cups of flour, salt, and mayonnaise to the bowl. Mix on low speed for about one minute to combine the ingredients thoroughly. Then, increase the speed to medium and mix for an additional 2 minutes. If you're mixing by hand, use a fork to blend the ingredients together until they are well combined.

3. Switch to a dough hook attachment if using a stand mixer, or prepare to knead by hand with intention. Gradually add the remaining cups of flour, one cup at a time, kneading gently as the dough absorbs it (If the dough is too loose, work in up to 2 additional cups of flour gradually, just until it comes together.) Once fully incorporated, stream in the melted, cooled butter slowly, letting it weave through the mixture like silk.

Continue kneading for 5 to 7 minutes, or until the dough becomes soft, elastic, and impossibly delicate, so light it clings like a whisper to your fingertips, almost pourable in its silkiness. This isn't just dough, it's the cloud in your bread's name taking shape.

4. Rest the Dough: Transfer the kneaded dough onto a clean, lightly floured surface. then gently fold the dough a few times to create surface tension. Prepare a large bowl (a wooden bowl is ideal) by adding a splash of olive oil or avocado oil to the bottom. Place the dough into the bowl, rolling it around to ensure the bottom is coated in oil. Flip the dough over so that the oiled side is facing up. Cover the bowl with a piece of plastic wrap and a kitchen towel, then place it in a warm spot to rise for about one hour, or until it has doubled in size.

5. Prepare for Baking: Once the dough has risen, line two baking trays with parchment paper to prevent sticking.

6. Shape the Buns: After the dough has doubled, transfer it to a clean, floured work surface. Divide the dough into 8 equal pieces. Take each piece, one at a time, and shape it into a ball. Gently flatten each ball to form a bun shape, and place them on the prepared baking trays, spacing them about two inches apart. If you're using two trays, distribute the buns evenly between them. Cover the trays with a kitchen towel and let the shaped buns rest for 25 minutes.

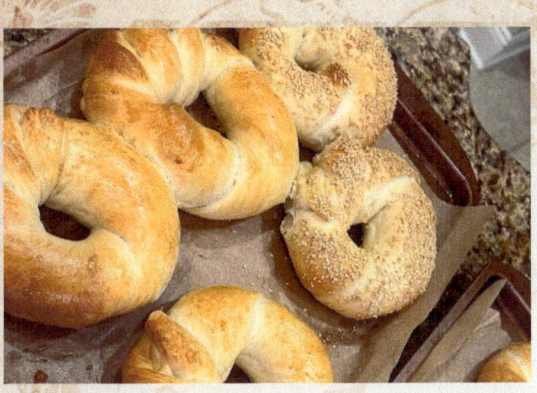
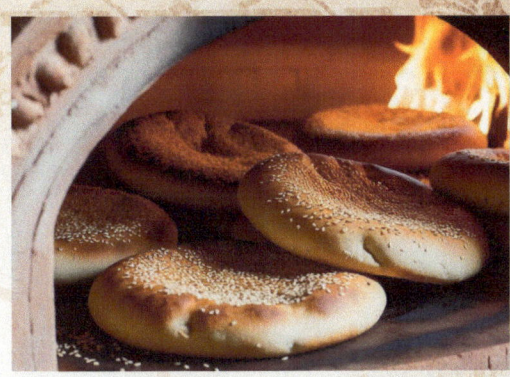

7. Prepare for Topping: Halfway through the resting period, preheat the oven to 450 degrees Fahrenheit. In a small bowl, crack and beat the egg until it's fully combined. When the buns have completed their resting time, uncover them and prepare for the next step. Using an Uzbek bread stamp, quickly make a decorative imprint in the center of each bun. If you don't have a stamp, you can use a fork creatively to create holes, just be sure to only poke in the middle.

8. Add Egg Wash and Seeds: With a kitchen brush, carefully apply the beaten egg all over the tops of the buns, ensuring an even coating for that beautiful golden finish. For a touch of flavor, sprinkle black seeds in the centers of each bun.

9. Create Steam and Bake: To enhance the texture of the bread, place a few ice cubes in each corner of the baking tray and underneath the baking sheet. This will create steam in the oven as the ice melts, contributing to a fluffier result. With everything ready, quickly place the trays in the preheated oven, ensuring that heat doesn't escape by closing the door promptly. As I always do, I remember my grandmother's wisdom about hot ovens being essential for excellent bread.

10. Bake to Perfection: Bake the buns for about 15 minutes, or until they turn a lovely golden brown and the bottom is light nice and bronze. Once they are done, remove the trays from the oven and allow the buns to cool on a wire rack before serving.

Freezing Tip: (3-6 months)

Got extra bread? No problem! Just let it chill out, then tuck it into freezer bags for a frosty nap in the freezer!

ENJOY THE DELIGHTFUL AROMA AND THE SATISFYING TASTE OF YOUR HOMEMADE BREAD!

Magnesium Spray
The Red Pill of Rest

I thought anemia was the fight. Iron pills, absorption charts, endless bottles lined up like soldiers. But the real battle wasn't iron at all. It was magnesium - or rather, the absence of it - quietly rewriting my body's code while I kept looking the other way.

Sleepless nights. Muscles wound tight like wire. A nervous system buzzing like static. That wasn't weakness. That was the system glitching.

The Awakening

You can swallow capsules forever and still feel empty. Because the truth is this: healing isn't about more. It's about access. About finding the doorway no one told you existed.

For me, that doorway was transdermal absorption. Magnesium sprayed onto the soles of the feet - minerals slipping past the gatekeepers of digestion, straight into the bloodstream. No detours. No wasted effort.

The first night, it hit like a reboot. Sleep didn't just arrive - it pulled me under. Muscles unclenched. Thoughts went silent. The system reset.

Why Magnesium Matters

- Grounding: Guides calcium into bone, steadies the heart's rhythm.
- Release: Dissolves tension in muscles that have carried too much for too long.
- Calm: Quiets the mind, slows the racing, restores balance to the nervous system.
- Truth: Shows you that deficiency isn't weakness - it's interference.

The Experience

Spray. Wait. Let the minerals sink in. The tingling is just the system waking up. The deeper gift is what follows: rest that feels earned, strength that feels inevitable, peace that feels like freedom.

Magnesium is the red pill. Once you experience it, you can't go back.

Moringa: The Green That Doesn't Even Go Here (But Runs the Place Anyway)

You know that belly chaos - the gas, the bloat, the heaviness that makes you feel like you swallowed a balloon animal? That's SIBO (Small Intestinal Bacterial Overgrowth) trying to sit at your lunch table. It's loud, messy, and refuses to leave.

Enter moringa. Not the polite, kale-adjacent leaf you sprinkle on a smoothie. No. This is the green that slams its tray down, stares SIBO in the face, and says: "You can't sit with us."

Why Moringa Is the Empress of Greens

- Protein Power Move: More protein per gram than yogurt. Dairy? You're officially irrelevant.
- Iron Throne: Out-irons spinach so hard Popeye would switch sides. Sorry, sailor.
- Vitamin C Flex: More than oranges, without the sugar crash. Citrus can go cry in the bathroom.
- SIBO Smackdown: With antimicrobial and anti-inflammatory compounds, moringa doesn't soothe belly bullies - it expels them.

How to Drink It Like You Own the Hallway

Boil 2 cups of water. Kill the heat. Stir in ½ teaspoon moringa powder. Add lemon if you're feeling extra. Sip it like the reigning queen of the cafeteria sipping her cranberry juice — smug, unbothered, untouchable.

The Experience

The first sip? Earthy, unapologetic, a little savage. But then it hits - cravings calm, belly lightens, energy steadies. Moringa doesn't whisper promises; it delivers receipts.

If your gut has been acting like a mean girl, moringa is the one who writes SIBO's name in the Burn Book with a single line: "She doesn't even go here."

When I compare myself to
the vastness of the Earth, I often feel incredibly small,
helpless, even, beneath its immense beauty and timeless
complexity. Standing under an expansive sky or gazing at
towering mountains, I begin to wonder: what impact can
a single dot of humanity have on such a magnificent
land? It's tempting to ask, "What can a tiny creature like
me possibly contribute to this grand tapestry of life?"

Yet as I pause and listen to the world around me, the
rustle of leaves, the breath in my chest, the quiet gift of
sunrise, I'm reminded of what Earth has already offered
me: its bountiful resources, its breathtaking landscapes,
and the rhythm of life itself. In that reflection, I find not
insignificance but uniqueness. My sense of worth begins
to shift, measured not by stature or possession, but by
how I perceive myself in this intricate web of existence.

Instead of waiting passively for others to initiate change,
I choose to act. I recognize the quiet power within me,
the ability to shape moments, influence lives, and leave
an imprint, however small, on the path I walk. It's a
strength born not from loud declarations but from
intentional steps.

This journey of self-discovery has revealed a simple truth:
I am the center of my own universe. Not in egotism, but
in awareness. With this realization, I rise above the
cacophony of doubt and fear, embracing my potential.
Each step I take (no matter how tiny) is a contribution to
the larger whole. And that
knowledge empowers me to walk this Earth with
purpose, humility, and
unwavering intention.

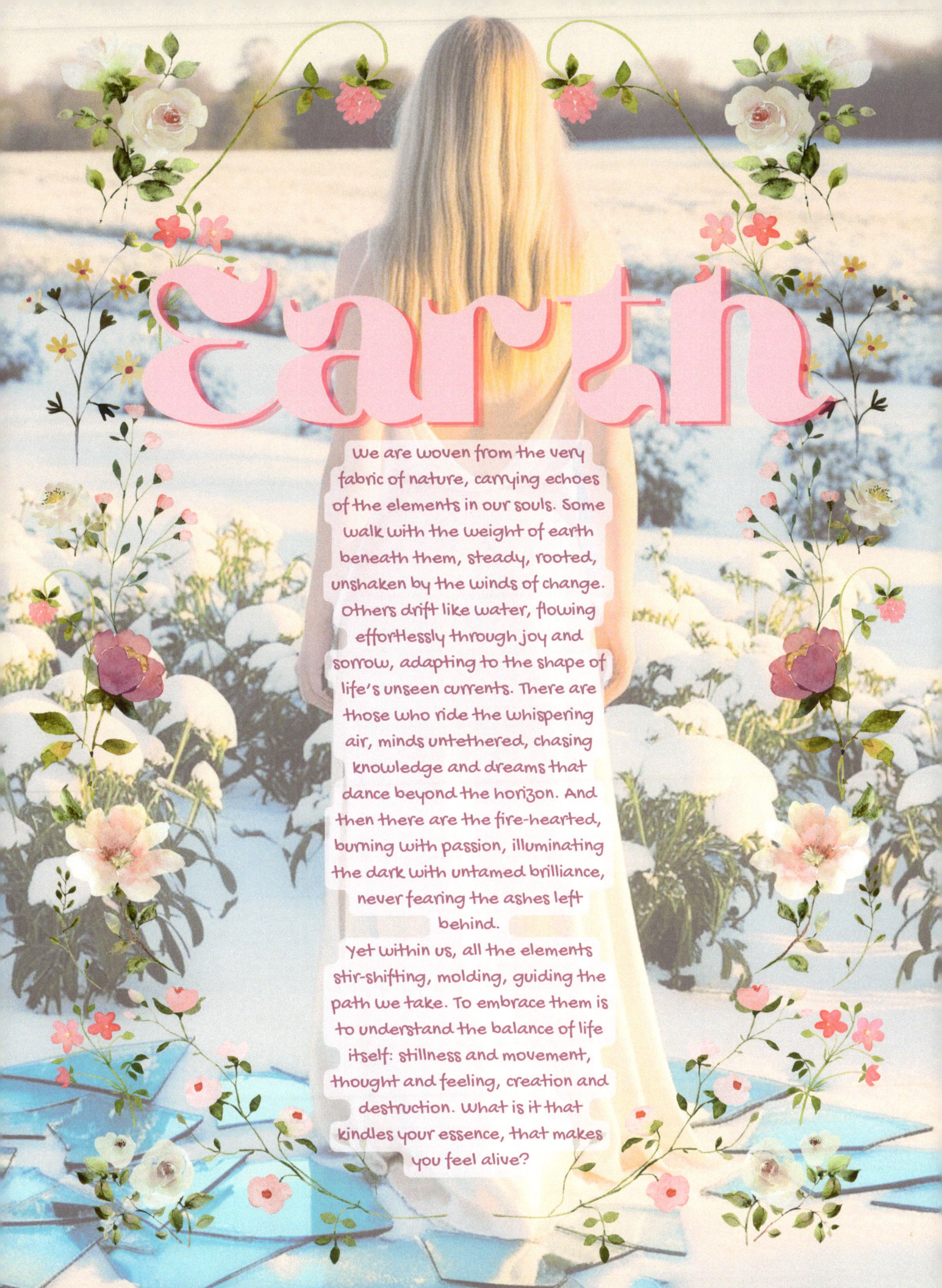

earth

We are woven from the very fabric of nature, carrying echoes of the elements in our souls. Some walk with the weight of earth beneath them, steady, rooted, unshaken by the winds of change. Others drift like water, flowing effortlessly through joy and sorrow, adapting to the shape of life's unseen currents. There are those who ride the whispering air, minds untethered, chasing knowledge and dreams that dance beyond the horizon. And then there are the fire-hearted, burning with passion, illuminating the dark with untamed brilliance, never fearing the ashes left behind.

Yet within us, all the elements stir-shifting, molding, guiding the path we take. To embrace them is to understand the balance of life itself: stillness and movement, thought and feeling, creation and destruction. What is it that kindles your essence, that makes you feel alive?

Connect

With Nature

earth

symbolizes stability and grounding, representing the firm foundation on which we walk and build our lives. Our connection to the Earth spans hundreds of thousands of years, illustrating a bond that is deeply rooted in our shared history. The Earth not only supports and envelops us but also nurtures our basic needs, providing shelter, materials for construction, and the resources necessary for survival. This element embodies the essence of the material world and our physical existence, highlighting the significance of practicality and nurturing in our daily lives.

The Earth is often associated with concepts of reliability and security, emphasizing the profound ties we have to our natural environment. It offers essential resources—such as food, water, and raw materials—that sustain us, reflecting our dependence on the land and its bounty. Moreover, Earth serves as the foundational bedrock of our existence, reinforcing a timeless sense of permanence, strength, and resilience.

The Earth nurtures our communities and shapes our homes, giving us a sense of belonging. It serves as a reminder of the importance of caring for the environment and recognizing our connection to all living things. By developing a deeper appreciation for the Earth, we can better understand our responsibilities toward it. This way, we can ensure that future generations will also enjoy the incredible present and presence of our planet.

Thoughts

Transform each day into a breathtaking masterpiece, fully embracing all its highs and lows.

Grounding

I have always felt a profound connection to the mountains, a bond that traces back to my childhood. Long car rides, where my only view was the majestic peaks stretching towards the sky, left a lasting impression on me. Those journeys were accompanied by the twinkling stars above and the enchanting stories my parents shared. They often spoke of the paries; winged female creatures of extraordinary beauty, resembling humans yet magical in nature. To add excitement and a touch of fear, they spun tales of jinn, mischievous spirits that would supposedly kidnap paries if they did not eat their meals. I can still recall the mix of wonder and laughter that enveloped me as I watched my siblings' eyes widen in fright, all while we gazed at the clear, starry skies, half-hoping to catch a glimpse of those enchanting beings.

Reflecting on my grounding practices, I've always felt that the mountains symbolize the earth's steadfastness. My curiosity about grounding grew as I learned about the benefits of connecting with the earth barefoot. Initially, the thought of feeling the various textures and potential bugs on the ground filled me with apprehension. However, over time, I embraced the experience and even found joy in it. Despite my initial fears, there is something incredibly liberating about loosening my grip on these worries. That said, my absolute favorite grounding experience occurs at the beach. There's a unique delight in feeling the wet sand beneath my bare feet as the waves gently lap at my ankles. When that cool water splashes against me, I can almost feel all the negativity and stress washing away, pulled deep into the earth. Each breath of salty air rejuvenates me, connecting me not just to the ground but to the vastness of nature itself. It's a reminder of the beauty and simplicity of existence, a true moment of peace amidst life's chaos.

Scientific research suggests that grounding can significantly reduce stress levels by lowering cortisol, improve sleep quality through enhanced circadian rhythms, and promote emotional stability by fostering a more balanced state of mind. The practice encourages a deeper awareness of bodily sensations and heightened mindfulness, leading to a more profound sense of tranquility and harmony.

By engaging in grounding, individuals can absorb the Earth's subtle electrical and magnetic energies, which helps to rejuvenate the body's physiological systems. This reconnection not only enhances physical vitality but also supports mental clarity, emotional regulation, and spiritual wellbeing. Grounding encourages us to cultivate a mindful relationship with our surroundings, appreciation for the intricate beauty of nature, and acknowledgment of the interconnectedness of all life. Ultimately, by grounding ourselves, we create a stronger, more resilient foundation for navigating the complexities of modern living, fostering a deeper sense of peace and fulfillment in our lives.

Planning *Thursday*

- *Feast Prep in Motion*

Kick things off by marinating chicken in tangy ranch - let the flavors sink deep so Thursday night dinner feels like a celebration. Add in mini samboosa, crisp and golden, stuffed with spiced veggies or meat. Bite-sized, irresistible, and guaranteed to impress.

- *Laundry Reset*

Clear the last loads, fold with intention, and stack everything neatly. Fresh, crisp clothes waiting in drawers? That's the kind of quiet win that makes the whole day smoother.

- *Deep Clean, Deep Refresh*

Vacuum every corner until the carpets show those satisfying lines. Wipe down baseboards, surfaces, and hidden spots - the kind of clean that makes the air itself feel lighter.

- *Glow Mode On*

Treat your skin to a face mask, then layer on your overnight care. By morning, you'll wake up looking and feeling renewed - Thursday night self-care that pays off in Friday confidence.

By the end of Thursday: the house is fresh, the food is prepped, the laundry is folded, and your skin is glowing. Productivity and pleasure, perfectly balanced

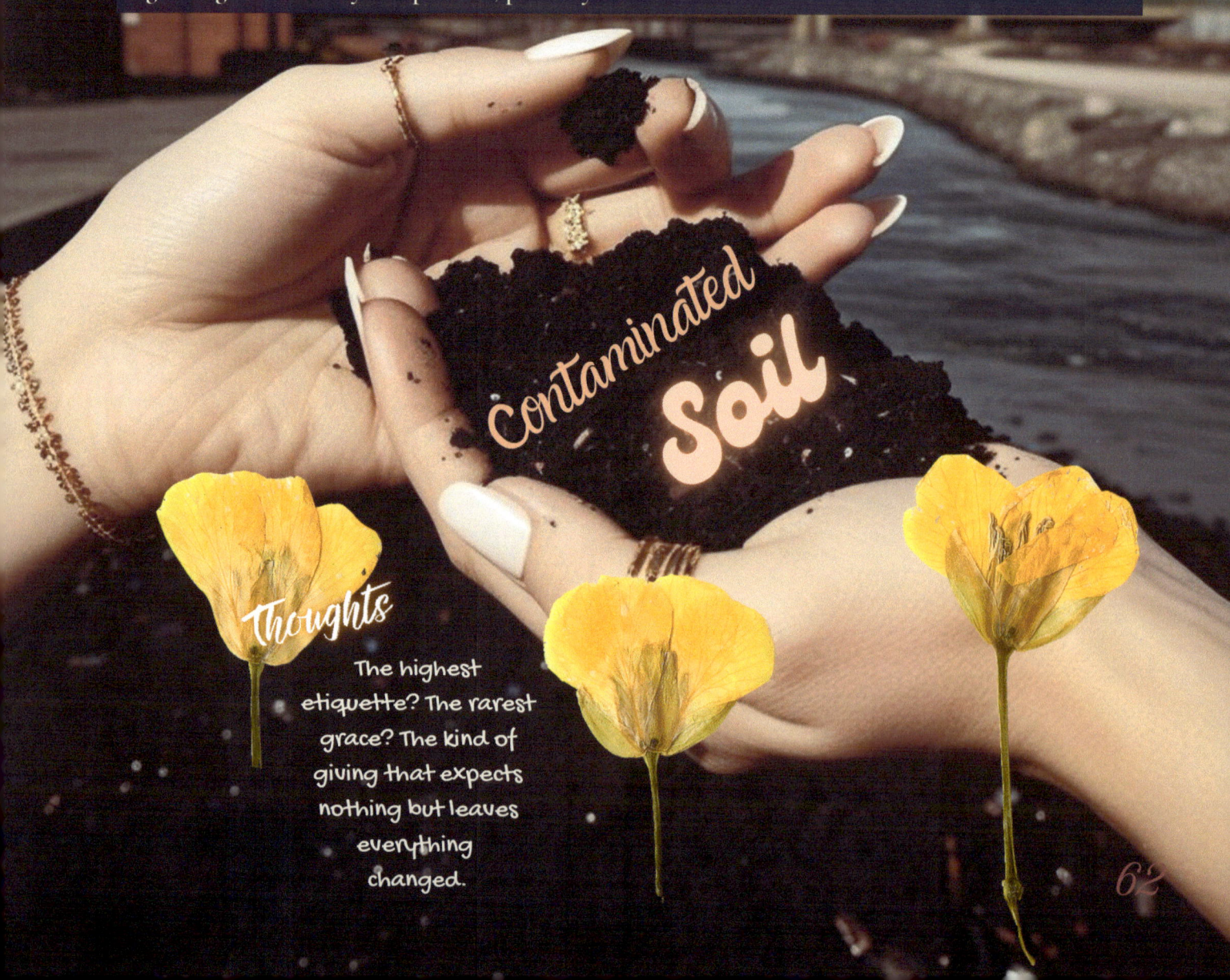

Contaminated Soil

Thoughts

The highest etiquette? The rarest grace? The kind of giving that expects nothing but leaves everything changed.

Soil: The Wound Beneath Our Feet

When I press my hands into the earth, I expect to feel life. Worms twisting, beetles darting, the quiet pulse of a living world. Instead, I feel betrayal. This soil - the very skin of the planet - carries poisons we poured into it. Heavy metals. Pesticides. Chemical ghosts that do not die. What should be sacred is scarred. What should feed us now threatens us.

This is not dirt. This is evidence. Evidence of our carelessness, our hunger for convenience, our refusal to see the cost. Every factory spill, every poisoned field, every careless runoff has left its fingerprint here. And the ground remembers. It remembers the toxins we buried, the ecosystems we dismantled, the life we silenced. And the cost is unbearable. Crops that no longer thrive. Rivers that run dirty. Insects vanishing, birds falling silent, forests thinning. Floods rising where roots once held the land. Even the climate itself unraveling, because soil - this quiet, overlooked ally - is one of Earth's great vaults of carbon. And when we wound it, it releases its storehouse like a scream.

Soil is not just a medium for plants. It is the hidden infrastructure of survival. A single teaspoon of healthy soil contains more microorganisms than there are people on Earth - bacteria, fungi, protozoa, nematodes - an invisible civilization that recycles nutrients, builds fertility, and keeps ecosystems alive. When we drench fields in chemicals, we don't just kill pests. We collapse entire underground cities. We erase the very engineers of life.

Soil is also water's keeper. It filters rainfall, recharges aquifers, and regulates floods. Strip it bare, compact it, poison it - and water no longer seeps down. It runs off, carrying toxins into rivers, fueling floods, leaving drought behind. What once was balance becomes chaos.

And soil is climate's quiet partner. It stores more carbon than the atmosphere and all vegetation combined. But when we plow recklessly, when we burn forests, when we leave land bare, that carbon escapes. The ground exhales centuries of storage in a single season, and the planet warms.
To hold soil today is to hold grief. It is to feel the weight of our undoing in the palm of your hand. And if that doesn't shake us, what will?
But grief is not the end. Soil remembers how to live. Beneath the scars, it still knows how to breathe, how to filter, how to cradle life. If we choose to restore it, it will rise again. Crops will return. Rivers will run clean. Species will find their way back. Even the climate will steady.

And the solutions are not mysteries. We know them. Regenerative farming that feeds the soil instead of stripping it. Cover crops that shield it from erosion. Compost and organic matter that rebuild its fertility. Wetlands restored, forests replanted, toxins banned. These are not dreams. They are choices.
This is not about gardening. This is not about nostalgia for green fields. This is survival. Soil is the foundation of food, of water, of air, of life itself. To ignore it is to surrender the future. To protect it is to fight for everything we love.

So let us kneel, not in despair, but in defiance. Let us press our hands into the wounded ground and vow: we will not let this living skin of the earth be lost. We will restore it. We will rescue it. Because saving soil is not an option. It is the rescue mission of our time.

Mini Sambosa

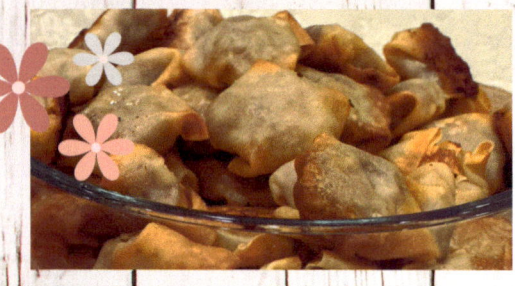

- 20 Good quality Egg Roll Wrappers 8"x8"
- One pound pasture-raised organic ground Beef
- One large Yellow Onion, thinly diced
- One teaspoon Salt
- ½ teaspoon ground black pepper
- ½ cup Avocado Oil

1. In a large mixing bowl, combine the ground beef, finely chopped onions, salt, pepper, and oil. Use your hands or a spatula to mix the ingredients until nicely combined.

2. Prepare a large baking sheet by lining it with baking paper.

3. Take 5 stacks of egg roll wrappers and carefully cut each stack in half lengthwise. Then, stack the resulting halves and cut them again in half widthwise, resulting in 20 small squares. Repeat this process with the remaining stacks of egg rolls until all wrappers are prepped.

4. Position one square of the egg roll wrapper on a clean surface. Place approximately half a tablespoon of the beef filling in the center of the square. Gently fold over the edges of the wrapper, pressing them together firmly to seal the filling inside; aim to avoid any exposure of the filling. Place the filled sambosa on the prepared baking sheet. Continue this process until all filling is used.

Freezing Tip: (*For future use, you can freeze the uncooked sambosas by arranging them on a baking sheet that fits your freezer. Once they are frozen solid, transfer them to freezer bags for storage. They can be kept frozen for up to a month.*)

5. About halfway through your filling process, preheat your oven to 375°F (190°C).

6. Once all sambosas are assembled, carefully place the baking sheet in the middle rack of the preheated oven. Bake for 15-17 minutes, or until the edges of the sambosas turn a delicious golden brown.

7. After baking, remove the sheet from the oven. Using a heat-resistant brush, lightly coat the tops of the hot sambosas with avocado oil for added flavor and a glossy finish. Let them cool for about 5 minutes before serving. Enjoy these delicious treats hot, or allow them to cool completely for future snacking!

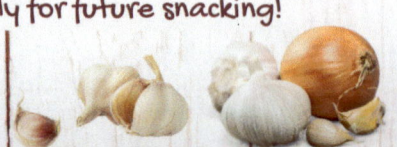

Garlic

My Ode to the Stinky Rose

When I first decided to explore garlic, yes, the so-called Stinky Rose, I thought I knew what I was getting into. Ancient cure-alls, vampire repellent, kitchen MVP. Cute. But the deeper I went, the more I realized: garlic isn't just a pantry essential, it's a full-blown superstar with layers (pun entirely intended).

Let's start with the drama. Garlic has been cultivated for thousands of years, think ancient Egypt, where it was so treasured they tucked cloves into tombs. (Tutankhamun, I see you.) In traditional Chinese medicine, it's considered a warming food used to push cold and damp out of the body, a spicy little bouncer for your immune system. And then there's allicin, the real magic that's unleashed the moment you crush or chop a clove. This spicy compound is garlic's calling card, loaded with antibacterial and antiviral powers that make it a one-bulb army against colds, flus, and general ickiness.

In folklore, garlic is often associated with warding off vampires and evil spirits, leading to its reputation as a protective herb. I clearly recall my second-grade experience of watching *Dracula* for the first time. My heart raced with both excitement and fear as I peeked out from behind the curtains, careful not to alert my parents. The chilling images sparked my imagination, and afterward, I embarked on a quest around the house to find garlic. I was determined to hang cloves in the windows, convinced that this age-old remedy would keep unwanted evening visitors at bay. Looking back, it brings a smile to my face, thinking about my innocent efforts to protect my cozy little world with a simple bulb.

But garlic doesn't just protect, it nourishes. One tiny clove packs a surprise punch of vitamin C, B6, calcium, magnesium, copper, potassium, and antioxidants. And it barely costs you any calories. Honestly, if garlic had a dating profile, it would be a total catch. Even better? Garlic has made its way into the quirkiest traditions. In some cultures, it's tucked into wedding ceremonies for luck, health, and a long, happy life. Imagine dancing into forever with your person, a clove tucked somewhere in the mix for good measure. Kind of amazing, right?

So whether you're tossing it into your favorite dish, wearing it like medieval armor against sniffles, or just admiring its unmatched charisma, let's be real: garlic is more than food. It's flavor. Folklore. Power. Prevention. And a whole lot of personality.

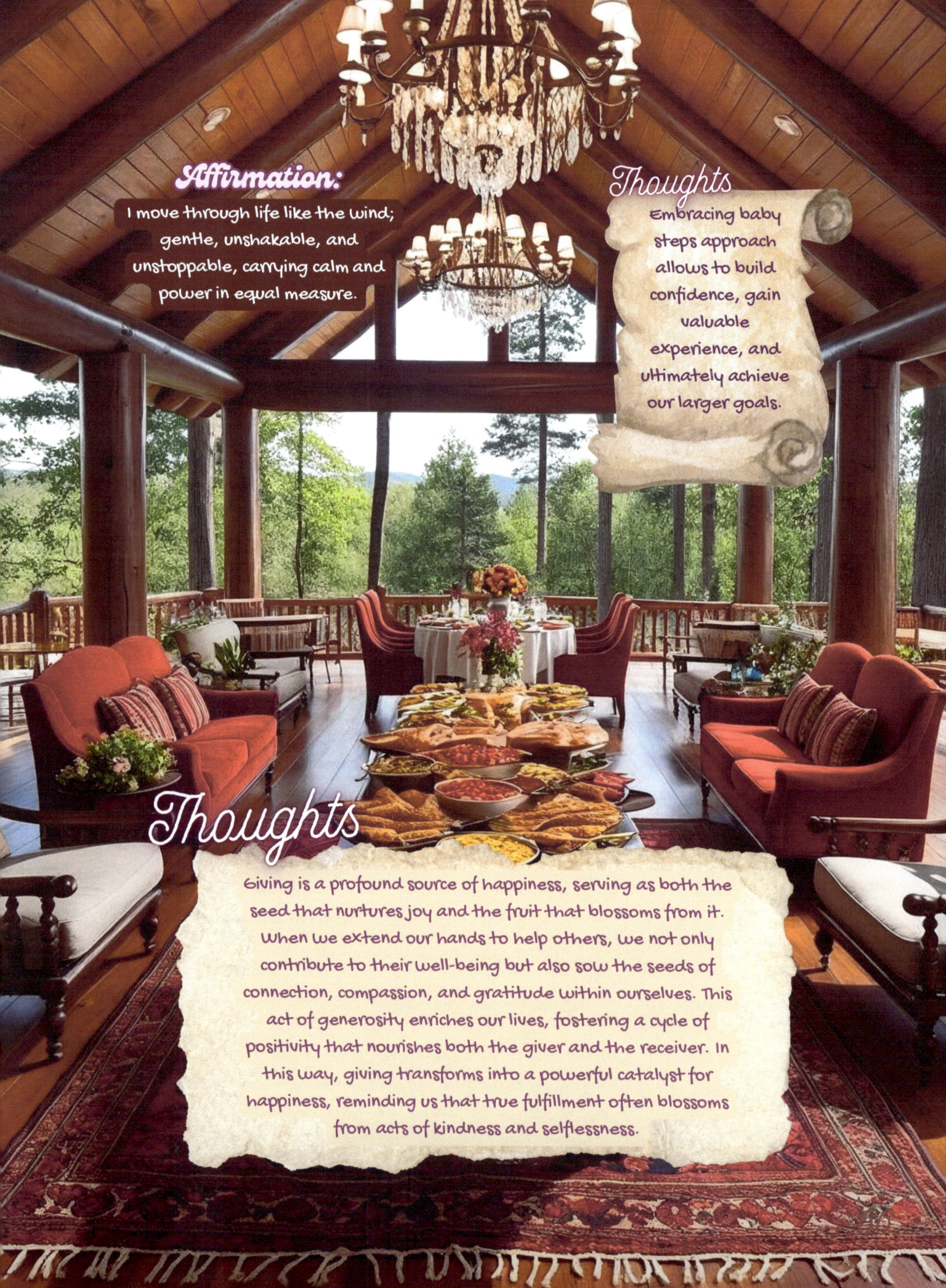

Affirmation:

I move through life like the wind; gentle, unshakable, and unstoppable, carrying calm and power in equal measure.

Thoughts

Embracing baby steps approach allows to build confidence, gain valuable experience, and ultimately achieve our larger goals.

Thoughts

Giving is a profound source of happiness, serving as both the seed that nurtures joy and the fruit that blossoms from it. When we extend our hands to help others, we not only contribute to their well-being but also sow the seeds of connection, compassion, and gratitude within ourselves. This act of generosity enriches our lives, fostering a cycle of positivity that nourishes both the giver and the receiver. In this way, giving transforms into a powerful catalyst for happiness, reminding us that true fulfillment often blossoms from acts of kindness and selflessness.

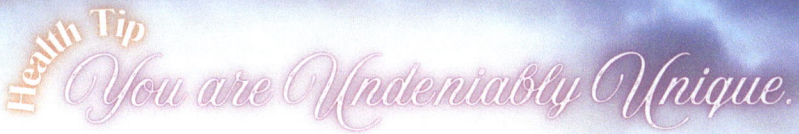

The Art of Health: A Journey as Unique as You

Your body is a story, an intricate, living narrative woven from the threads of ancestry, environment, and the choices you make each day. No two people share the same biological fingerprint, which is why wellness cannot be reduced to a formula. The concept of bio-individuality reminds us that health is not about following someone else's path, but about embracing our own. It's about listening to the quiet signals of our bodies, to the echoes of our past, and to the deep wisdom that tells us what we truly need.

The Echoes of Ancestry: Love, Legacy, and the Lessons We Carry

Health is more than science; it is tradition, memory, and love. The foods that nourished our ancestors, the bread baked with care, the spices passed down through generations, become a part of us, shaping not just our physical selves but our emotional ties to nourishment. But the connection runs deeper. Epigenetics, the study of how environmental factors influence gene expression, tells us that our lifestyle choices don't just affect us; they can alter the way future generations experience health. If generations before us embraced certain foods or habits, their presence lingers in our preferences and struggles. A grandmother's love for rustic bread might make abandoning carbs feel like severing a generational bond. Likewise, the shadow of past addictions can manifest in cravings, despite the conscious knowledge of their harm.
Even before birth, a mother's emotions, diet, and stress levels subtly imprint upon her child's developing nervous system, leaving whispers of love in every cell.

One Size Doesn't Fit All: The Beauty of Personalized Nutrition

Health is not a checklist. It is an ever-evolving relationship, with food, with movement, with ourselves. No universal diet or lifestyle can capture the magic of individuality. Metabolic diversity means that some people thrive on low-carb diets, while others need complex carbohydrates for energy. Even gut microbiomes, the billions of microorganisms that play a role in digestion and immunity, vary significantly from person to person, influencing how foods are processed and absorbed. True wellness is found in self-trust, the willingness to experiment, adapt, and listen with care. It is the kind of love that asks, What do I need today? rather than demanding rigid perfection. And when we nourish ourselves with understanding rather than pressure, we don't just gain health, we gain peace.

The Evolving Path to Optimal Well-Being

Health is a love story, a lifelong dance between what we know and what we discover.
It shifts with time, with seasons, with the rhythm of our lives. The nervous system adapts, hormones fluctuate, and even our microbiome evolves based on what we eat, how we move, and the emotions we experience. The journey to well-being is not about arriving at an endpoint; it is about growing, learning, and embracing the constant act of becoming. There is beauty in the search, grace in the imperfections, and deep joy in the simple act of honoring who we are, uniquely, wonderfully, and unapologetically.

Onion Bread

Thoughts

Capture the vibrant moments of joy, the little details of daily life, and even the challenges that shape our experiences.

Let's make Onion Bread

If you are a true fan of flavorful breads, you will undoubtedly fall head over heels for this captivating onion bread, which I affectionately refer to as Piyazlik Na'an in Uzbek. While it may not be a staple in every bakery, it holds a special place in my heart and kitchen.

The experience of enjoying this bread takes on a whole new dimension when paired with creamy, tangy cream cheese the following day, it's truly a match made in gastronomic heaven!

Crafting this delightful bread is a breeze. Begin by using the same dough recipe that you would for a Uzbek bread. Right before you place it in the oven, incorporate thinly sliced one large red onions, tossed lightly in flour to help absorb moisture and enhance the bread's texture. For a bit of heat, add some freshly chopped jalapeños to the mix.

Once all the ingredients are thoroughly combined, spread the dough evenly onto a large, well-greased baking sheet. Proceed with the remaining steps of your bread recipe, and before you know it, your home will be filled with the tantalizing aroma of baking bread. Prepare to enjoy bread that's not only delicious but unforgettable! Enjoy every wholesome slice!

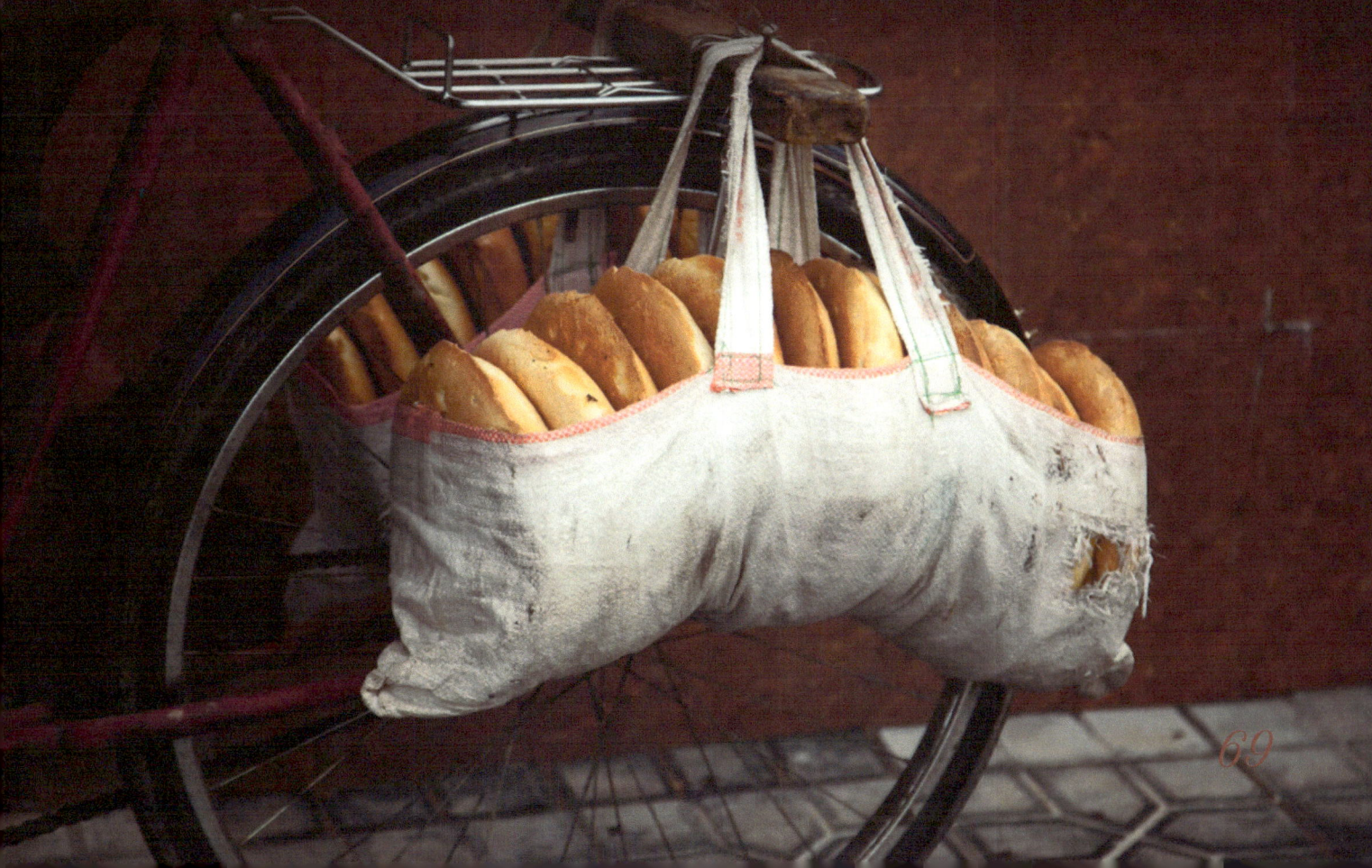

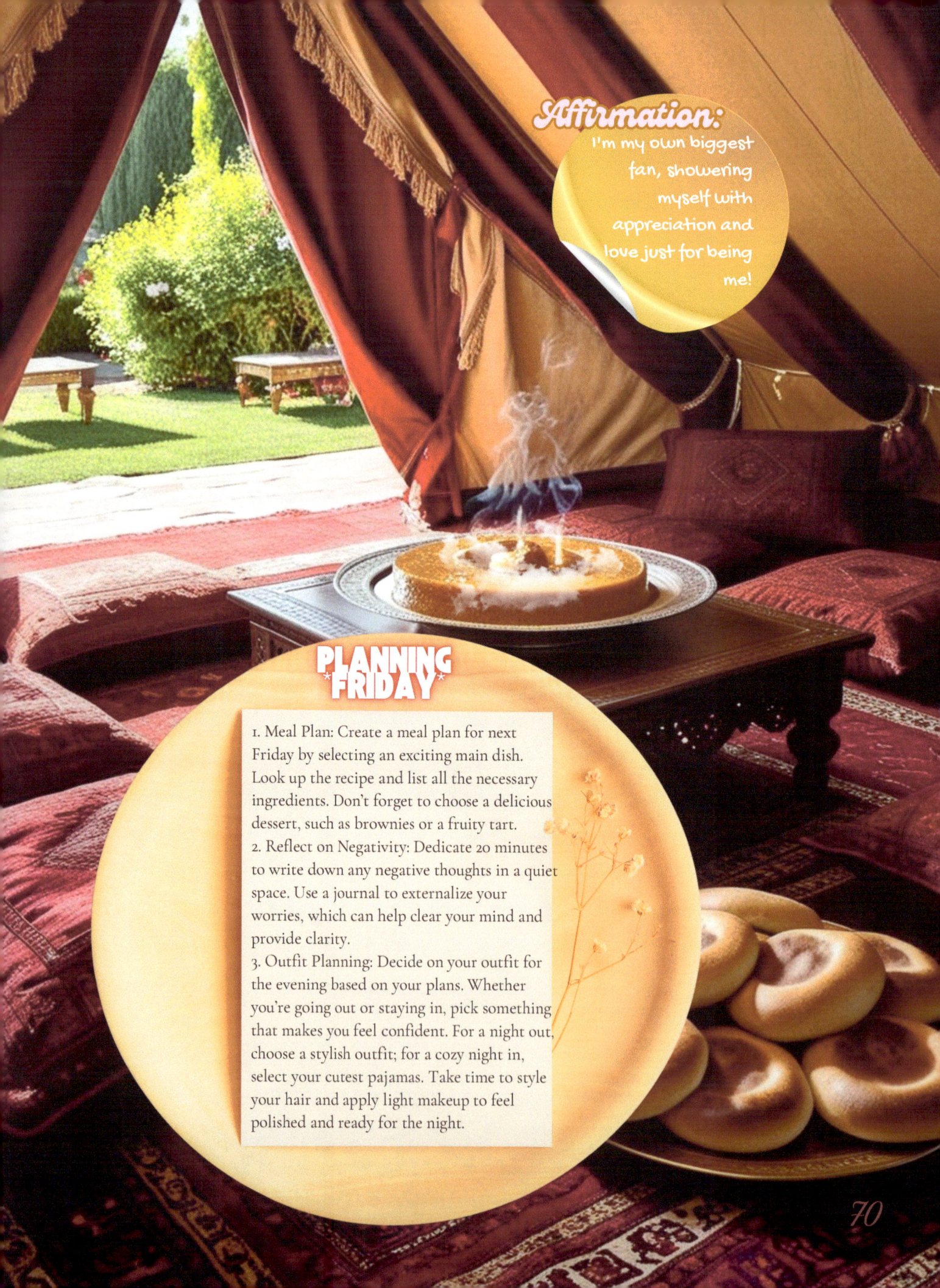

PLANNING *FRIDAY*

1. Meal Plan: Create a meal plan for next Friday by selecting an exciting main dish. Look up the recipe and list all the necessary ingredients. Don't forget to choose a delicious dessert, such as brownies or a fruity tart.

2. Reflect on Negativity: Dedicate 20 minutes to write down any negative thoughts in a quiet space. Use a journal to externalize your worries, which can help clear your mind and provide clarity.

3. Outfit Planning: Decide on your outfit for the evening based on your plans. Whether you're going out or staying in, pick something that makes you feel confident. For a night out, choose a stylish outfit; for a cozy night in, select your cutest pajamas. Take time to style your hair and apply light makeup to feel polished and ready for the night.

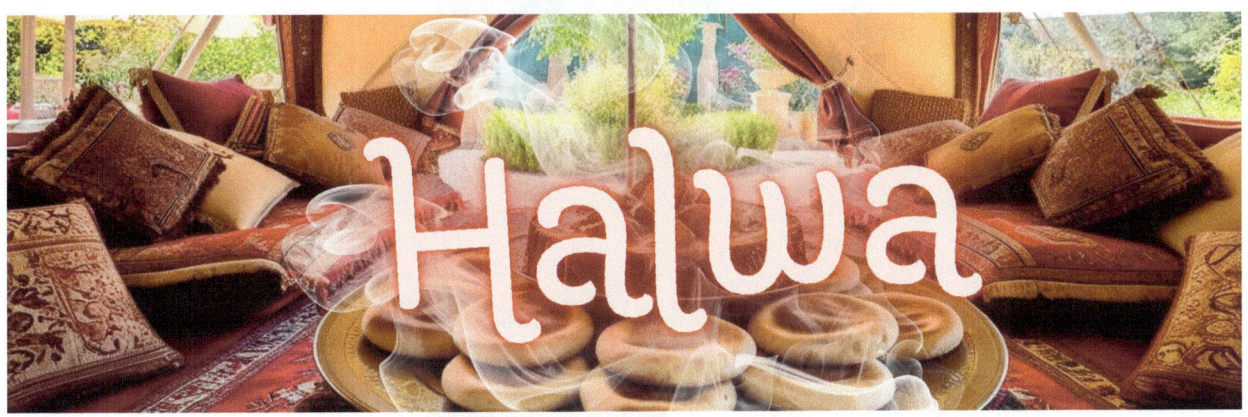

Halwa

Halwa is a delightful and simple sweet dish that has deep cultural roots in Uzbek, Afghan, Indian, and Arab cuisines. Its significance extends beyond mere culinary pleasure; it is often intertwined with religious traditions and celebrations. I was sitting in a small French bakery with a dear Greek friend, sipping coffee and sharing macarons, when I showed her this part of the book. She looked at the word halwa on the page, then said softly, "We have it too. We spell it halva." And something in me stilled. We were surrounded by polished pastries and Parisian charm, yet suddenly I was back in my mother's kitchen, and she was in hers. Different languages, different kitchens, but the same sweetness. It felt like my mother's glassy halwa had quietly walked across a continent and found a second home. I hadn't expected that. But she saw it, felt it, claimed it. And in that moment, I realized this wasn't just a dish—it was a bridge. A small, sacred one. The kind you don't build, but find.

My mother used to prepare various kinds of halwa, each with its own unique flavor and texture. Some of her favorites included those made with wheat, besan (gram flour), carrots, and my personal favorite, sheeshaye halwa, which translates to "glassy halwa."

I remember the old tales about halwa: in our culture, there was a superstition that if someone asked for halwa and it wasn't made, it would be a sign of impending misfortune, even death. As a child, I found this concept amusing. I would eagerly request the glassy halwa, the most challenging version to make, and my mother, despite her busy house chores, would often get annoyed. Yet, she would always end up putting everything aside to prepare it for me. This made me feel special, even though I knew it was a labor-intensive treat.

Despite my fond memories, I must admit that I've never quite mastered the recipe myself. Halwa has always been one of those elusive dishes: sometimes it would turn out perfectly, while other times, it would be a complete failure. I recall vividly the sight of my mother making a large pot of halwa, filling the kitchen with its aromatic sweetness. Afterward, she would create small sandwiches using pita bread, lovingly wrapping them before distributing them to the less fortunate who gathered outside the holy mosque in Madina after Friday prayers. I would assist her in this act of kindness, and those moments spent handing out food to those in need left an indelible mark on my heart—it was a blend of warmth, community, and gratitude that I cherish to this day.

Halwa was pure joy; a little tradition, a little mischief, and a whole lot of love. My mother would sigh, then smile, then work her magic, turning my pleas into the sweetest indulgence. Every bite tasted like love, patience, and happiness wrapped in sugar.

Some recipes, however, are not meant to be written down—they live in the hands that stir the pot, in the scent that fills a home, in the shared laughter over a simmering stove. My mother's halwa was exactly that: something that could not be captured in mere words or measurements. Perhaps that's why the recipe isn't in this book. Or perhaps, deep down, I still believe that if I ever try to write it down, I'll never quite get it right the way she did.

And so, halwa remains a story, a tale of love, persistence, and generosity—sweet enough to linger on the tongue and in the heart forever.

Simit

Simit is a Turkish bread shaped like a ring and covered in sesame. The crust is crisp, the inside is soft and chewy, and the sesame hits first-nutty, toasty, loud. You tear it, not slice it. It's usually handed over warm, wrapped in thin paper, still steaming from the stall. One bite and you get it: this bread doesn't need toppings, but it plays well with jam. Especially the kind I keep in my fridge.

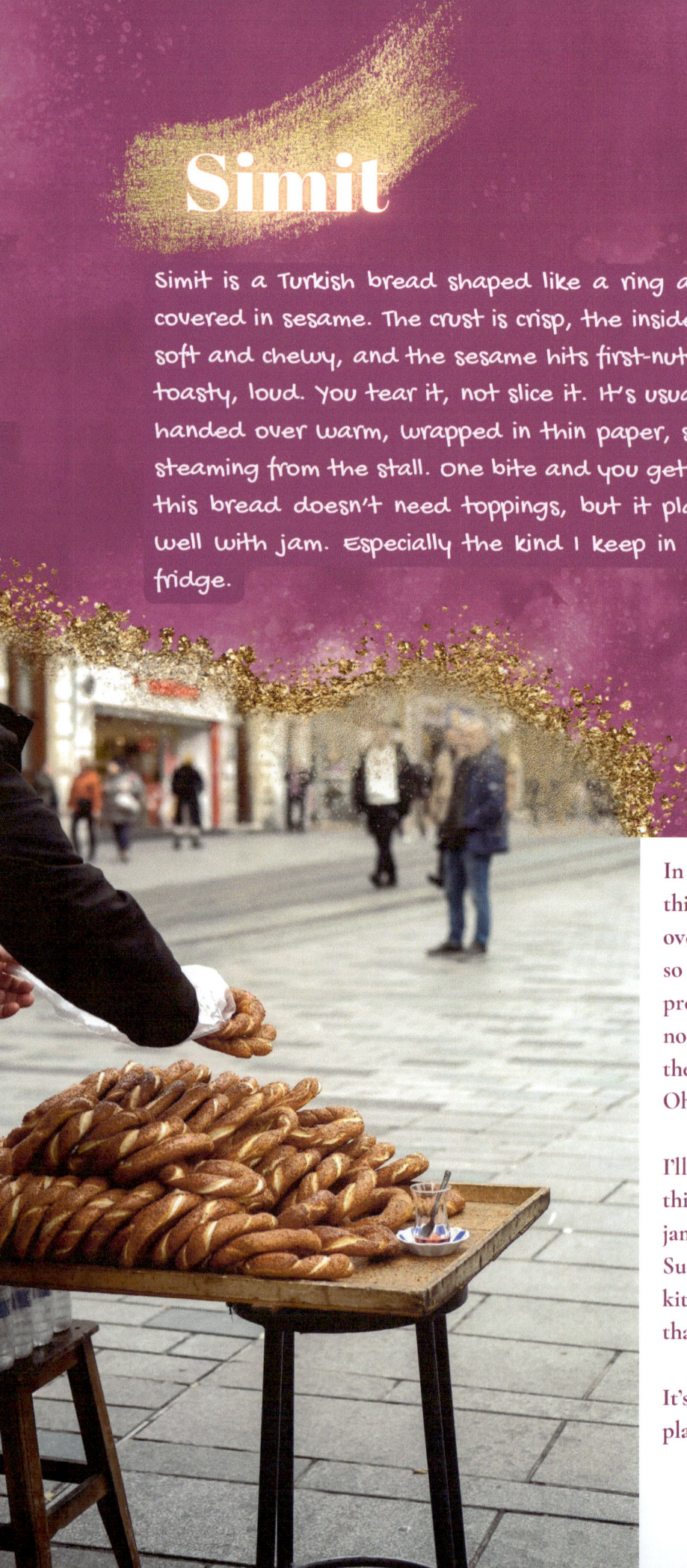

In Uzbek culture, guests bring bread. It's a thing. A beautiful, generous, slightly overwhelming thing. Sometimes they bring so much, I start stacking loaves like I'm prepping for a carb apocalypse. I smile, I nod, I say "how lovely," and I mean it... in theory. But if I spot simit in the mix? Oh. My. Day. Is. Made.

I'll sneak it to the side, wait for the crowd to thin, then pull out my mother's homemade jams like I'm unlocking a secret level. Suddenly there's an after-party in the kitchen; just me, a few chosen guests, and that perfect, sesame-studded circle.

It's not just bread. It's the one that gets a plate, a story, and a seat at the table.

Let's make Simit

I'll guide you through making simit bread using my Uzbek bread recipe, to step 5. (p53-55)

1. **Prepare the Dough:** Begin with your prepared dough. Once it has doubled in size—a sign that it's ready, carefully transfer it to a clean work surface generously coated with melted butter. The butter not only prevents sticking but also adds a lovely flavor to the bread.

2. **Divide the Dough:** Using a sharp knife or dough cutter, divide the dough into 12 equal pieces. After cutting, cover these pieces lightly with a kitchen towel to prevent them from drying out while you work.

3. **Shape the Pieces:** Take two pieces of dough at a time and, using your oiled hands, roll each piece into a long strip about 10 inches in length. This process is quite enjoyable and will make you feel like a skilled, old-school chef! Utilize a gentle rolling and pulling technique to ensure the dough stretches evenly.

4. **Create the Twist:** Once you have both pieces rolled out, pinch the ends of each strip together to secure them. Then, twist the two strands around each other, forming a long, braided shape. Pinch both ends again to bring them together, shaping the twist into a circular form, resembling a bagel.

5. **Prepare the Coating:** In a medium-sized bowl, combine ¼ cup of pomegranate molasses with ¼ cup of water and a pinch of flour. Stir this mixture until it's well blended. In a separate shallow bowl, place 1 ½ cups of toasted organic sesame seeds, which will provide a delicious crunch and nutty flavor to your simit.

6. **Coat the Dough:** Take each twisted circle of dough and dip it into the molasses mixture, ensuring that you coat both sides thoroughly. After that, gently place the circle in the bowl of sesame seeds, again making sure that both sides are well-covered.

7. **Prepare for Baking:** Line a baking tray with parchment paper to prevent sticking. Place each coated simit on the tray, leaving about 2 inches of space between each one to allow for proper expansion during baking. Cover the tray with a kitchen towel and let the simits rest for 25 minutes. This resting period is crucial for the texture of the bread.

8. **Preheat the Oven:** About halfway through the resting time, preheat your oven to 400 degrees Fahrenheit.

9. **Bake the Simit:** Once the resting period is complete and your oven is preheated, carefully place the tray in the oven and bake the Simit for 15 to 17 minutes, or until they are beautifully golden brown. Once the baked goods have cooled to room temperature, transfer them to a wire rack to allow for proper air circulation. This will help prevent any moisture buildup and maintain their texture. Once cooled completely, enjoy the delicious treats! To keep them fresh, store the items in an airtight container at room temperature. They will stay delightful for up to four days. Enjoy each bite!

Keep in Mind
BABY STEPS

Each brushstroke of emotion adds depth and richness to the canvas of your existence, creating a beautiful extension that tells your unique story.

Thoughts

Affirmation:

I have the confidence to engage with others effectively, understanding that each interaction is an opportunity for growth and connection.

Tahini & Date Syrup
DIP:

This dip offers a satisfying experience that rivals the comfort of visiting your favorite coffee shop. It's particularly amazing when paired with fresh Simit bread and a steaming cup of dark Turkish tea, making for a perfect snack or light meal.

To create this very simple dip, start by taking a cute small flat bowl that showcases its international flair. Pour 4 to 5 tablespoons of high-quality creamy Tahini in the bowl then drizzle an equal amount of date syrup over the Tahini. The sweetness of the syrup wonderfully complements the nutty taste of the Tahini, creating an adventurous blend. Don't hesitate to get creative with your presentation; you could swirl the two together for an artistic touch or sprinkle some sesame seeds, cinnamon, or chopped nuts on top for added flavor and texture.

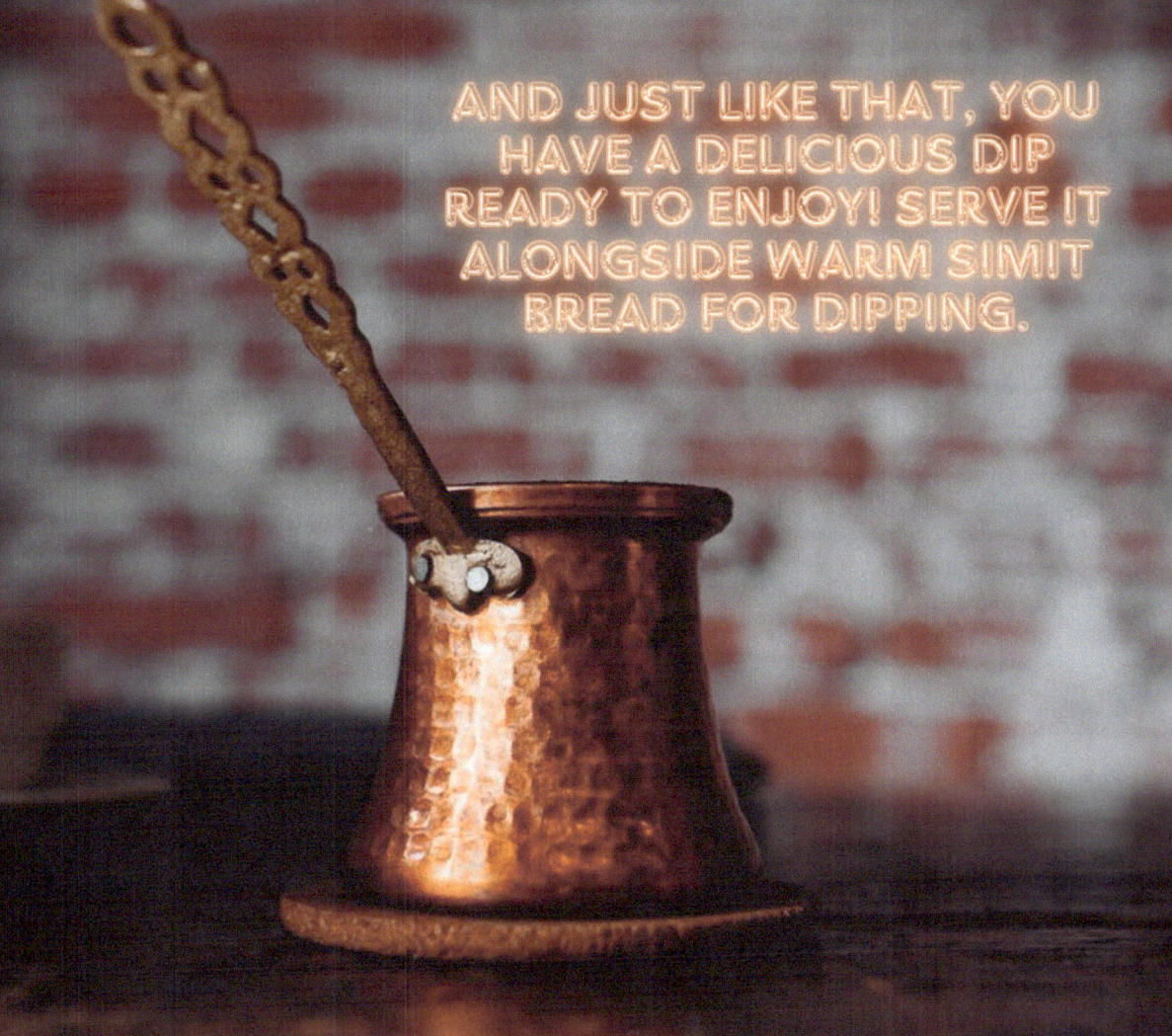

AND JUST LIKE THAT, YOU HAVE A DELICIOUS DIP READY TO ENJOY! SERVE IT ALONGSIDE WARM SIMIT BREAD FOR DIPPING.

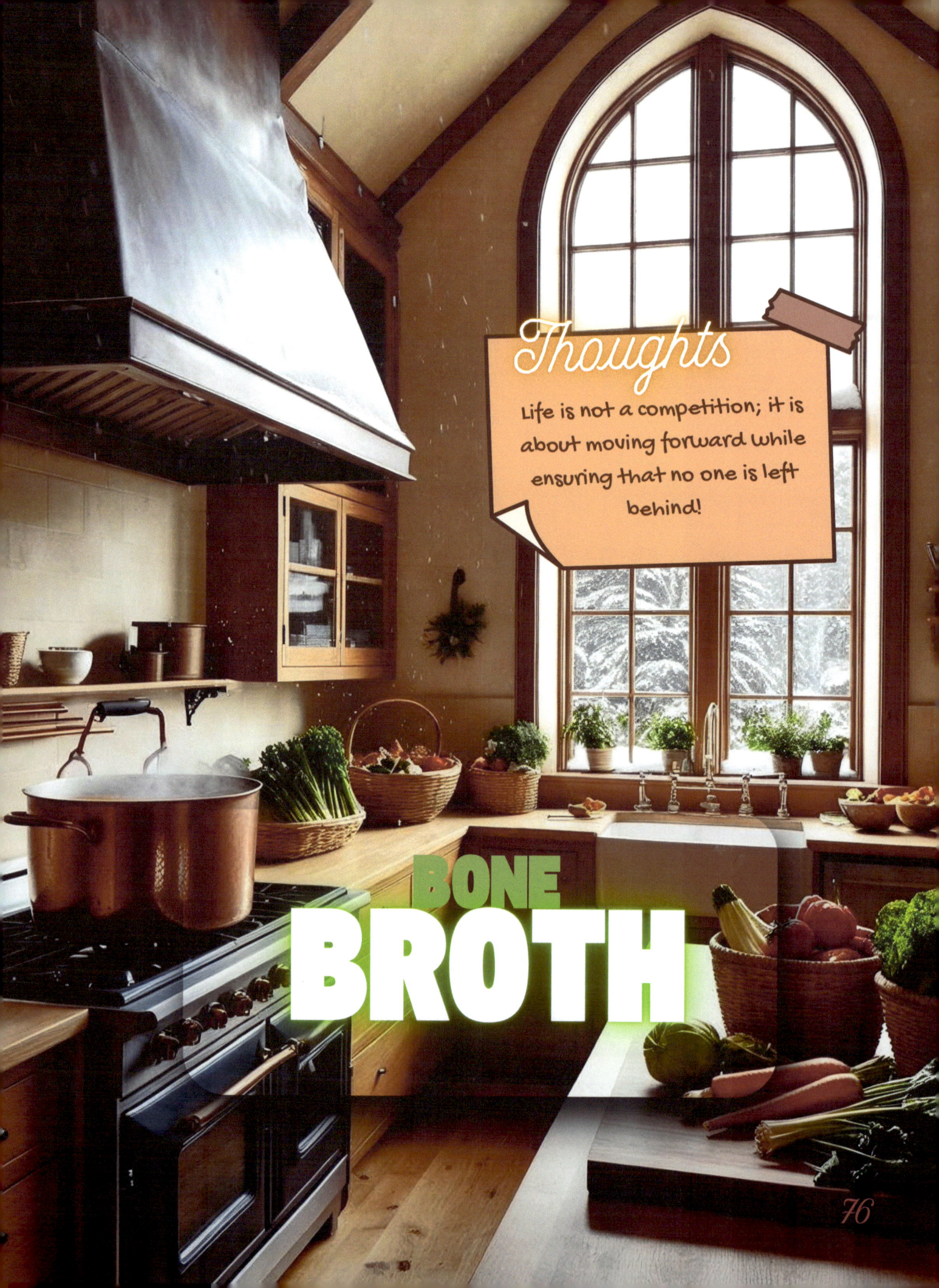

Thoughts

Life is not a competition; it is about moving forward while ensuring that no one is left behind!

BONE BROTH

LET'S EXPLORE THE WONDERS OF BONE BROTH

Bone broth, aka the "miracle drink," the "golden elixir," or just "BB" if you're tight on time, has been slurped up by cultures all over the globe for eons, thanks to its superhero-level health perks. Crafted by letting bones and connective tissues take a long, luxurious soak for over 12 hours, this nutrient-packed potion isn't just a tasty boost to your meals-it's a wellness whirlwind in a bowl!

One of the standout components of bone broth is collagen, a vital structural protein prevalent in skin, cartilage, and bones. Collagen has gained attention for its potential anti-aging properties, as it supports skin elasticity and hydration, potentially reducing the appearance of wrinkles. Moreover, as we age, our natural collagen production declines, making bone broth a valuable dietary supplement for maintaining youthful skin.

Beyond its beauty benefits, bone broth is revered for its role in digestive health. The gelatin derived from collagen helps soothe the gut lining, making it beneficial for individuals with digestive disorders such as irritable bowel syndrome (IBS) or leaky gut syndrome. Additionally, the amino acids found in bone broth, such as glycine and proline, play a crucial role in promoting digestive enzymes and supporting overall gut function.

From an immune support perspective, bone broth contains minerals like calcium, magnesium, and phosphorus, which are essential for maintaining optimal immune function. The warm, nourishing quality of the broth can also help alleviate symptoms associated with colds and flu, serving as a comforting remedy during illness.

Furthermore, bone broth is celebrated for its ability to promote joint health. The glucosamine and chondroitin found in bones are vital for maintaining cartilage integrity, which may help reduce symptoms of arthritis and joint pain. Many individuals consume bone broth as a natural way to support their active lifestyles and enhance recovery post-exercise.

Sleep is another area where bone broth shines. The presence of glycine not only promotes relaxation but also aids in improving sleep quality. Many people have reported that incorporating bone broth into their evening routine has led to better rest and overall well-being.

Over the years, numerous anecdotal accounts have surfaced, with many individuals crediting their experience with bone broth for a variety of health improvements. These include enhanced hormone balance, better digestive health, skin radiance, improved thyroid function, successful weight management, and even relief from allergies. The growing popularity of bone broth in wellness communities is a testament to its widespread recognition as a holistic remedy for enhancing overall health and vitality.

In a nutshell, bone broth isn't just a cozy cup of goodness; it's a nutrient-packed jackpot for your health! Whether you're sipping it solo, jazzing up soups, or sneaking it into smoothies, adding bone broth to your menu could be the tasty ticket to a healthier and more fabulous life.

How to Make Bone Broth Rich in Gelatin

Creating a delicious and nutrient-dense bone broth that is rich in gelatin requires attention to sourcing quality bones and using the right cooking techniques. Here's a detailed guide to help you achieve the perfect gelatin-rich broth:

Ingredients

1. Bones: I personally like beef bones. Look for joints, knuckles, and marrow bones, as they contain a higher concentration of collagen. Organic and grass-fed options are ideal for better flavor and nutritional profile.
2. Water: Use filtered water for the best taste.
3. Acid: Add a tablespoon of apple cider vinegar or lemon juice to help extract minerals and collagen from the bones.
4. Vegetables: Include aromatic vegetables such as onions, carrots, and celery for additional flavor. Herbs like parsley, thyme, and bay leaves can also enhance the broth.
5. Spices (optional): Consider adding peppercorns or garlic for extra depth of flavor.

Tips for Success

- For an even richer gelatin content, use a higher ratio of joints and connective tissues to meat.
- If the broth does not gel once cooled, it may not have cooked long enough, or the type of bones used may not contain sufficient collagen.

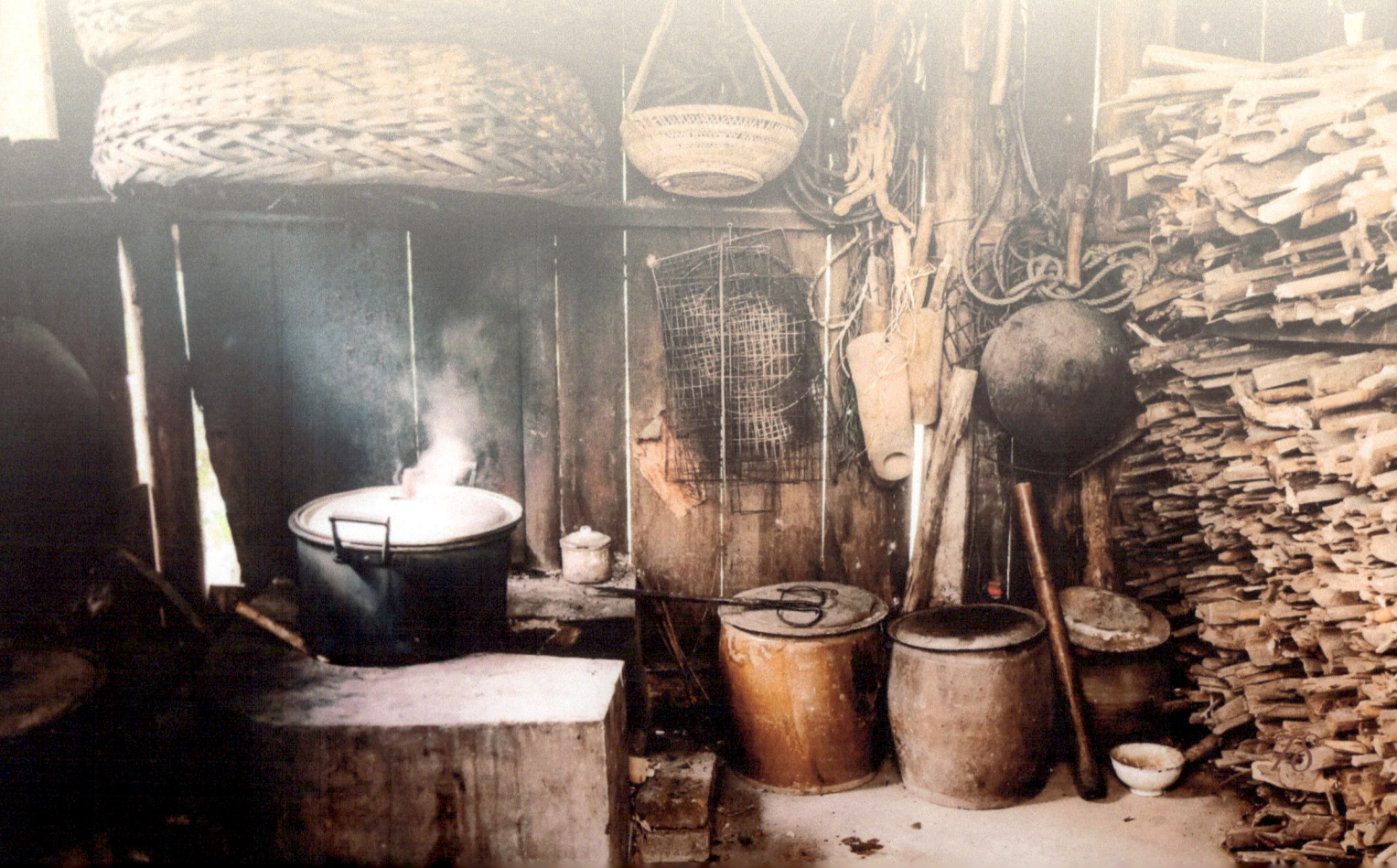

1. Preparation of Bones:
If using raw bones, you can roast them in the oven at 400°F (200°C) for 30-40 minutes to enhance the flavor. This step is especially beneficial for beef bones.

2. Combine Ingredients:
In a large pressure cooker, combine your prepared bones, chopped vegetables, and any herbs or spices.
Pour in enough filtered water to cover the ingredients completely, leaving about an inch of space at the top.

3. Add Acid:
Add a tablespoon of apple cider vinegar or lemon juice to the pot. This will help break down the collagen and increase the gelatin content in the broth.

4. Cooking Process:
Make sure to meticulously follow every instruction provided with your pressure cooker to ensure optimal results. Set the cooking time for 6 hours. Alternatively, if you prefer to use a deep saucepan, you can achieve a similar outcome by cooking on low heat for approximately 12 hours, allowing the flavors to develop fully. Once the designated cooking time has elapsed, carefully release the pressure according to your pressure cooker's guidelines. This often involves using a long utensil to avoid steam burns and ensuring that the lid is opened slowly and away from your face.

6. Straining:
Once cooked, strain the broth through a fine-mesh sieve or cheesecloth to remove the solids. Allow the broth to cool before transferring it to containers.

7. Storage:
You can store the broth in mason jars in the refrigerator for up to a week. If you're looking to keep it for longer, consider freezing it in smaller portions. Just a little tip when you freeze, make sure to leave some space in the jars for expansion. I know how disappointing it can be to find a jar has broken in the freezer.

How to Make Bone Broth Rich in Gelatin

Chicken Soup

My mother had a way of noticing the small failures in a body before anyone else did. She did not rush to prescriptions as a default; she moved instead toward the kitchen, toward the slow work of making something that would sit on the chest like a promise. Her instincts were practical and exacting, taught by years of watching people mend: a boiled chicken that smelled like home, a pot that hummed on the back burner, a ladle that arrived before words had finished falling apart.

Once, when I was twelve and fever-clouded, she stood over the stove and told me about the purple turnip, how the older women in our family swore by it because it cleared the chest in stubborn ways that salt and steam alone could not. She talked as she stirred, not to be mysterious but to teach me how care looks and sounds: "You do not bribe an illness; you invite it to leave by making the body want to stay whole." Her voice was steady; the soup was louder than the worry.

I learned from watching her choose the pieces that mattered: thighs kept in the freezer for speed, a knot of ginger for clarity, a handful of turnips because she trusted the old promise. She never dismissed modern medicine; she simply believed another kind of medicine lived in bowls and heat and the ritual of being tended. When antibiotics were necessary, she never argued; when they were not, she offered a different answer-one that smelled like garlic and held like a blanket.

Her generosity was not sentimental. It was disciplined. She browned the chicken like a small act of defiance against fatigue, let the onion soften until it smelled like patience, and added the turnip at just the moment it could do the most good. While the pot simmered, she sat with the sick person, a watchful quiet that kept panic from filling the room. Her presence turned a kitchen into a clinic and a bowl into proof that someone was staying.

The soup she taught me to make is simple, but its backbone is stubborn love. It taught me how to show up when the world prefers to look away. It taught me that tending is a verb, not a sentiment, that the truest medicine is often the steady repetition of small, exacting acts.

If you want the recipe, it's on the next page. For now, keep this: when you are called to care, bring heat, bring patience, and bring something unexpected-a purple turnip, perhaps-and let the bowl say what words cannot.

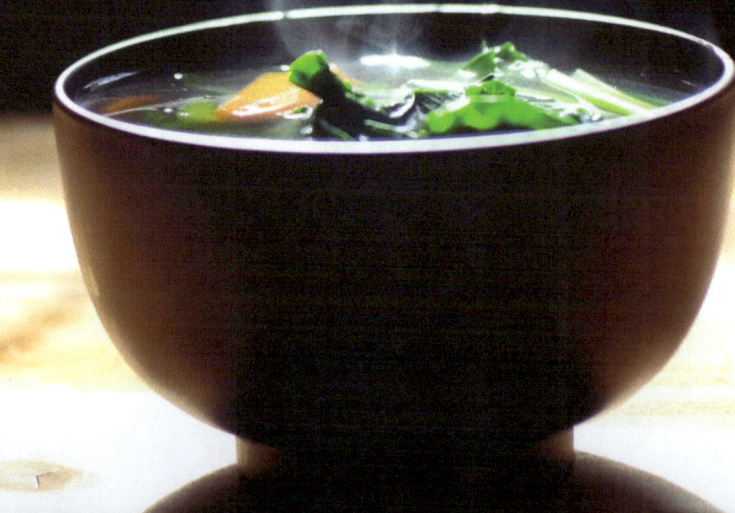

Ingredients:

- Four pieces of organic chicken thighs (or any bone-in chicken parts)
- One large Onion
- One peeled Whole Carrot
- 2-3 stalks of organic Celery
- One Purple Turnip, peeled and diced into half-inch cubes
- One teaspoon of organic Vegetable Boullion
- One teaspoon of organic turmeric powder
- One teaspoon of ground black pepper
- ½ teaspoon of organic ginger powder
- Sprinkle of ground cloves
- ½ cup of fresh chopped dill or 1 teaspoon of dried dill (optional)
- 8 cups of filtered water
- One cup of organic 2 ingredients noodles of your choice.

Instructions:

- Begin by gathering all the ingredients for your soup and place them in a large soup pot, with the exception of the noodles. Carefully pour in hot water until the ingredients are submerged, then add a generous sprinkle of salt to enhance the flavors. Bring the mixture to a boil over medium-high heat, then reduce the heat to low and allow it to simmer gently for about one hour.

- Once the hour is up, use a slotted spoon to carefully remove the onion, celery, and carrot from the pot, discarding. Next, gently lift out the chicken pieces, taking care not to break them apart in the process. Allow the chicken to cool for a few moments before starting to separate the meat from the bones. Use your hands or a fork to shred the meat into bite-sized pieces, and make sure to dispose of all the bones. I find that my cat, little Leo, enjoys the slimy bits and joints, so I give those to him as a treat.

- With the chicken set aside, it's time to add the noodles to the bubbling broth. Cook them according to the package instructions, but keep an eye on the clock. Four minutes before the noodles are fully cooked, stir in the shredded chicken to allow it to warm through and absorb some of the delicious broth.

- For an extra touch of flavor, sprinkle some dried mint from your pantry into the pot. Finally, serve the soup warm, garnished with a dash of fresh lemon juice for brightness.

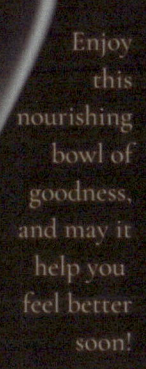

Enjoy this nourishing bowl of goodness, and may it help you feel better soon!

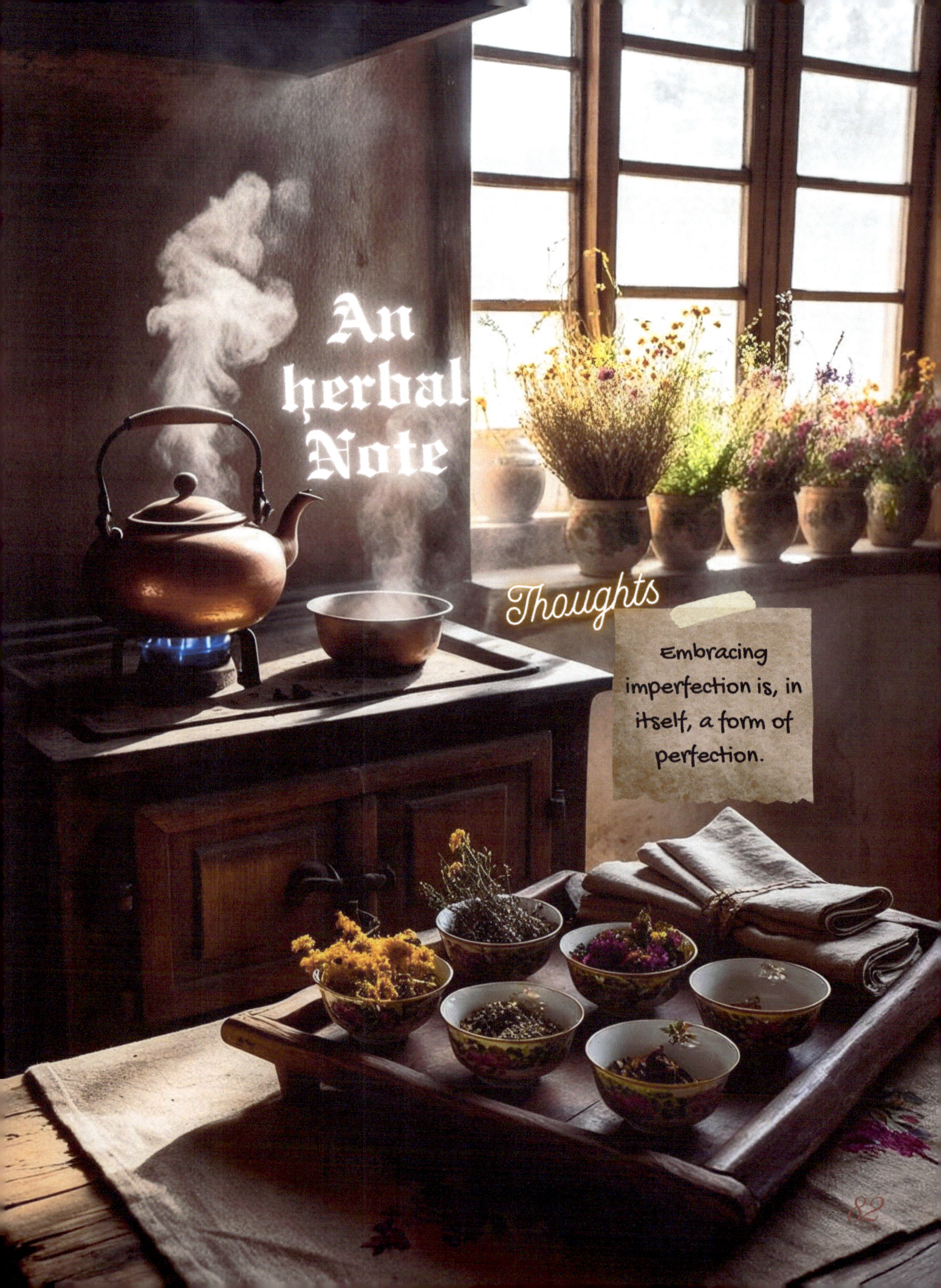

An herbal Note

Thoughts

Embracing imperfection is, in itself, a form of perfection.

The journey began when one of my children fell ill and required surgery, a process that stretched over several months. During that time, I remained resolute and kept my emotions in check, focusing entirely on supporting my child. Once the ordeal was over and my child had recovered, however, the stress took a toll on my own health.

I have struggled with anemia throughout my life, but the additional strain from the situation, coupled with hormonal imbalances, caused my cortisol levels to skyrocket. This resulted in an unexpectedly heavy and persistent monthly cycle, further exacerbating my anemia and posing serious health risks.

In an attempt to regain some stability, my doctor prescribed progesterone medication. While it initially helped alleviate the heavy cycles, I soon found that my body did not react well to the medication. I experienced intense episodes of heart palpitations at night, leaving me feeling as if my heart might give out. Ultimately, I made the decision to stop the medication.

In search of a natural remedy, I researched alternatives and discovered that fenugreek seeds could provide some relief. With caution, I decided to try them out. On the first day of taking the seeds, I noticed a gradual improvement, and by the third day of consuming them once daily, my heavy cycle was substantially reduced.

While fenugreek showed promise in balancing my hormones, I encountered other side effects as well. I noticed an unwanted increase in weight and an unpleasant body odor that made me reconsider my usage. For now, I've decided to use fenugreek only as needed, recognizing its potential benefits while remaining mindful of my body's responses. Fenugreek truly has numerous advantages, and I'm grateful to have discovered it during this challenging time.

Fenugreek is known for its remarkable benefits in promoting hormonal balance. This herb contains compounds such as phytoestrogens that may mimic estrogen in the body, which can be particularly beneficial for women experiencing hormonal fluctuations during menopause or menstruation. Additionally, fenugreek may help regulate insulin levels, contributing to better metabolic function and improved reproductive health. Its rich content of vitamins, minerals, and antioxidants further supports overall hormonal health by reducing inflammation and promoting a balanced endocrine system. Incorporating fenugreek into your diet, whether through seeds, supplements, or teas, may foster a more stable hormonal environment and enhance overall well-being.

Stay Safe: Check with Your Doctor First Fenugreek is generally considered unsafe for pregnant women due to its potential to stimulate uterine contractions, which could lead to complications. It is essential to consult with your healthcare provider before using fenugreek, especially if you have pre-existing health conditions or are taking other medications. Always prioritize your health and discuss any herbal supplements with your doctor to ensure they are appropriate for your individual circumstances.

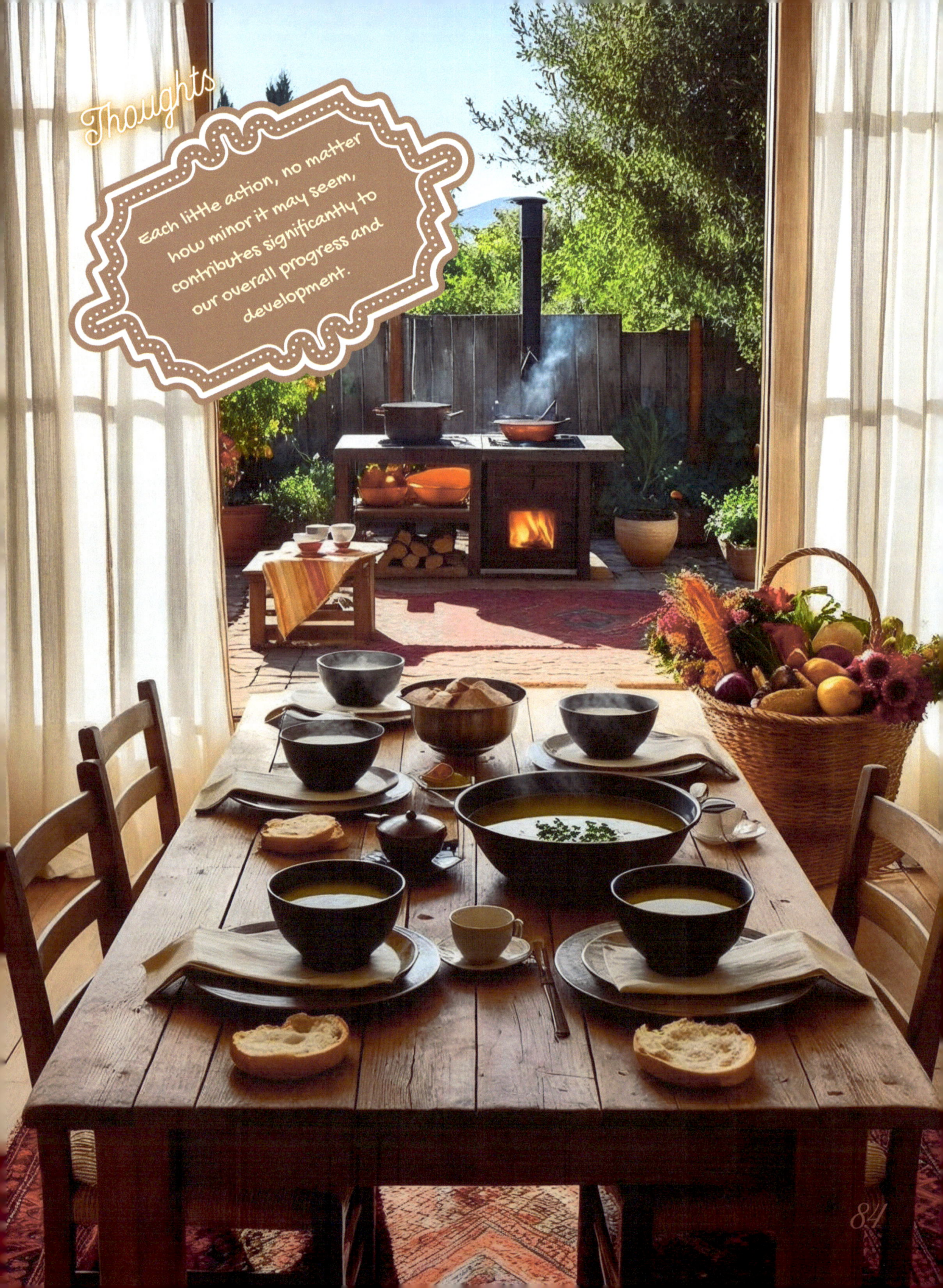

Each little action, no matter how minor it may seem, contributes significantly to our overall progress and development.

RICE
Spatula

In my life, rich with traditions and cultural heritage, the practice of collecting a dowry is seen as both a cultural and religious imperative when a girl is preparing to marry. This dowry typically serves to furnish the bride's future home with essential household items, referred to as Jaiz (Jihaz in Arabic and jahiz in Indian culture). These essentials include kitchen supplies, elegantly designed bed linens, luxurious blankets for the bedroom, and exquisitely crafted dishes for the dining room.

Conversely, the husband holds the responsibility for providing the residence itself and the furniture that adorns it. Among the items I received as part of my dowry, one particularly stands out: a bread press. This charming wooden tool, adorned with decorative nails, is used to create beautiful patterns on homemade bread, transforming a simple staple into a work of art. Additionally, I acquired a rice spatula, also known as a skimmer spoon, which is essential for preparing perfectly cooked rice—a staple in our cuisine.

Initially, I found these culturally significant items amusing, as they seemed to reduce the essence of womanhood to domestic responsibilities like bread and rice-making.

However as I journeyed through life, I began to understand the deeper wisdom embedded in these traditions. They reflect a profound respect for the art of homemaking, highlighting the vital role of nurturing and sustaining a family through skillful preparation and presentation of food. This realization has allowed me to appreciate the history and cultural significance of these seemingly simple tools, recognizing them as symbols of love and care that transcend generations.

UZBEK RICE

Uzbek rice is a dish that embodies simplicity yet demands meticulous attention to detail. The ingredients are straightforward, but mastering the technique can take time, and practice makes perfect. Traditionally, this rice is prepared using beef fat, which adds depth and richness to the final dish. Each grain of rice should be evenly coated with oil, a process that not only enhances flavor but also showcases your culinary skills —an aspect sure to impress even the most discerning traditional grandmothers.

One invaluable insight I gained from my father when he opened an Uzbek restaurant as a side venture was the significant role of the onion in achieving that perfect color for the rice. The secret lies in how the onion is prepared; it should be finely sliced and allowed to caramelize thoroughly. The rich golden hue of well-cooked onions infuses the rice with beautiful coloration and a subtle sweetness that elevates the dish.

Once you've perfected the art of making Uzbek rice, it can easily become a staple meal in your household, sure to delight family and friends alike. With each attempt, you'll find yourself improving and discovering new layers that make this dish uniquely yours.

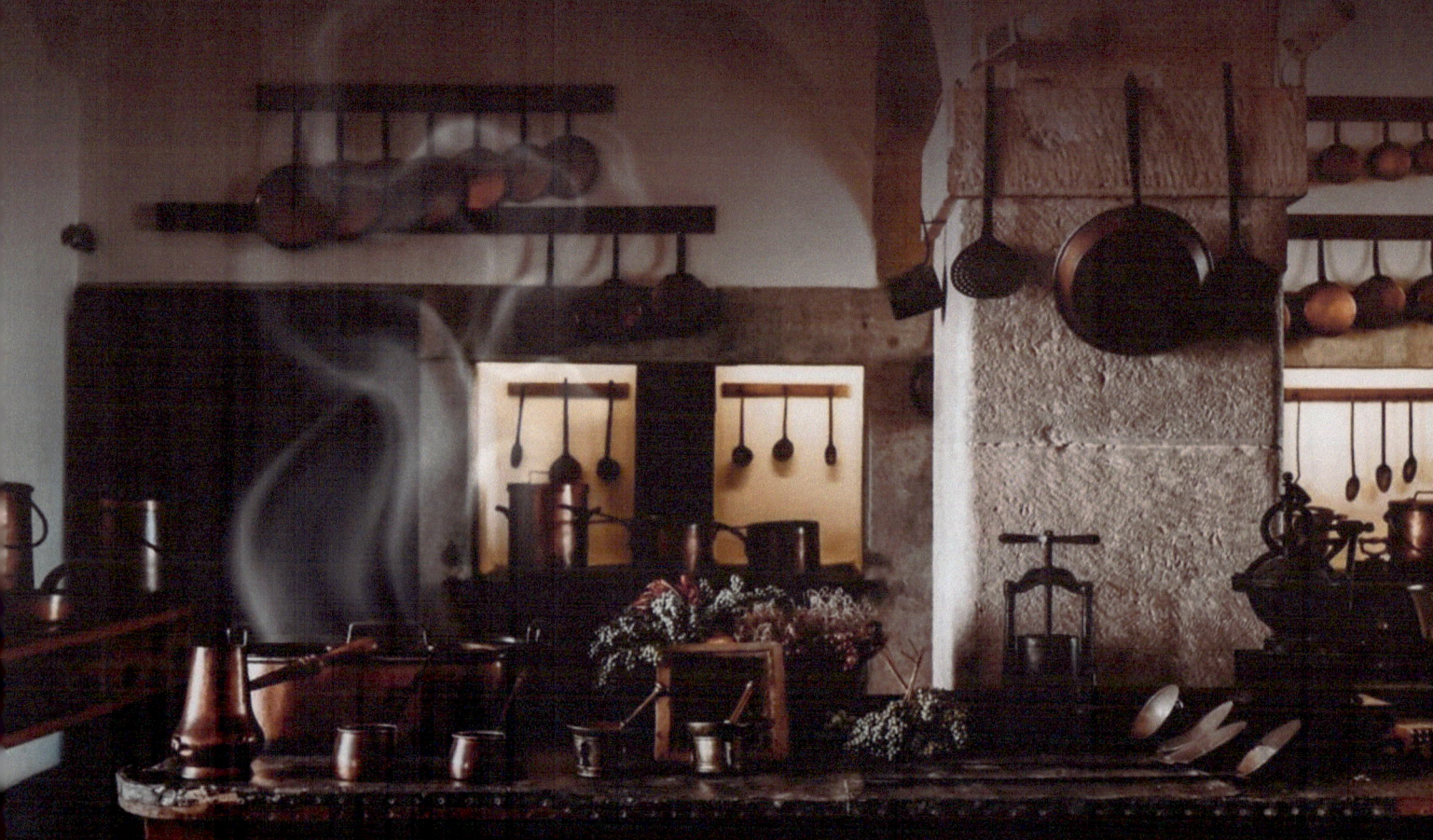

LET'S MAKE UZBEK RICE

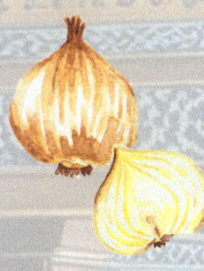

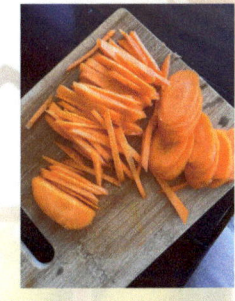

one cup of **Avocado Oil** extra for carrots & raisin

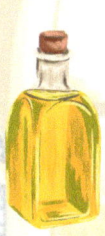

two Onions thinly sliced

one organic tomato chopped

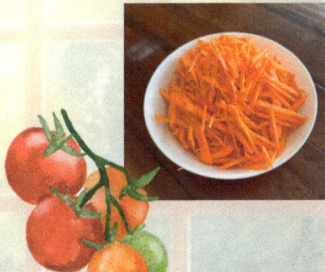

one tsp salt
one tsp ground black pepper
one tbsp ground Cuman

One pound of Beef with some bone and fat Cut into two inch cubes

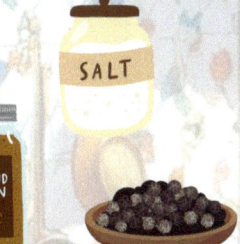

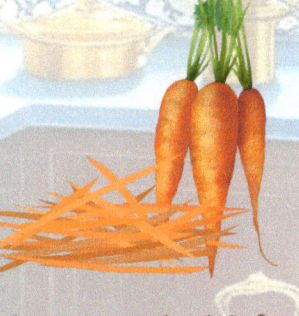

three peeled & j julienne carrots

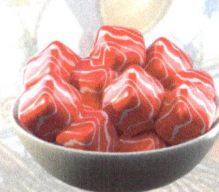

1/2 cup black Raisin

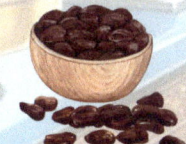

Rice Spatula

four cups Basmati Rice washed & soaked in cold filtered water for 2 hours

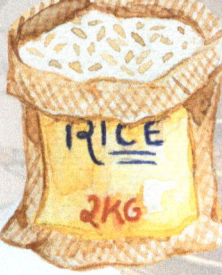

Instructions:

1. Begin by preheating a large, heavy-bottom stainless steel pot or a cast aluminum Kazan over medium heat for about one minute. Add avocado oil and allow it to heat for an additional minute. Once the oil is shimmering, add the thinly sliced onions, and immediately cover the pot with a lid. Ensure that the kitchen fan is on to prevent any lingering odors.

2. After five minutes on low heat, uncover the pot and increase the heat to medium-high. Stir the onions occasionally as they sauté, keeping a close watch on their color; this crucial step will determine the final hue of your rice, whether it achieves a winter pale or summer tan. Once the onions are perfectly caramelized, with a golden-brown central core and lightly browned edges, it's time to introduce your meat.

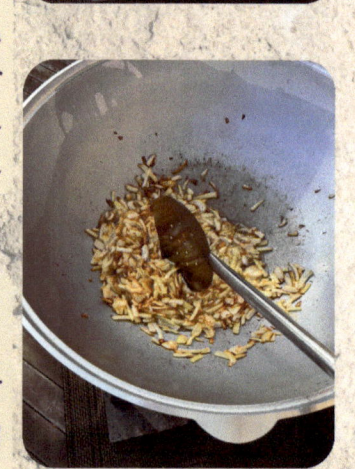

3. Add the meat to the pot, stirring to coat it evenly with the oil and onions. Season with salt and freshly cracked black pepper. Be mindful not to stir too vigorously; allowing the meat to sear slightly without overcrowding gives it a beautiful color. After a couple of minutes, add half of the julienne carrots along with a teaspoon of cumin, continuing to stir gently.

4. After 2-3 minutes, incorporate the diced tomatoes into the mix. Let them dehydrate on high heat for a few minutes to build flavor. Once the tomatoes are softened, add water to the pot, bringing it to a rolling boil. Then lower the heat to medium-low, partially covering the pot, and allow it to simmer for about an hour, or until the meat is tender and cooked through. A helpful tip from my mom: when the oil rises to the surface, it's a sign that the dish is ready for the next step.

5. While the meat is cooking, take a separate flat pan and heat up some oil. Sauté the remaining carrots for 5-7 minutes until they begin to soften. Once they reach the desired doneness, push them to one side of the pan and add the raisins, coating them lightly with oil without mixing them with the carrots. This technique enhances the flavors individually. For added sweetness, sprinkle the raisins with half a teaspoon of sugar, cover the pan, and turn off the heat.

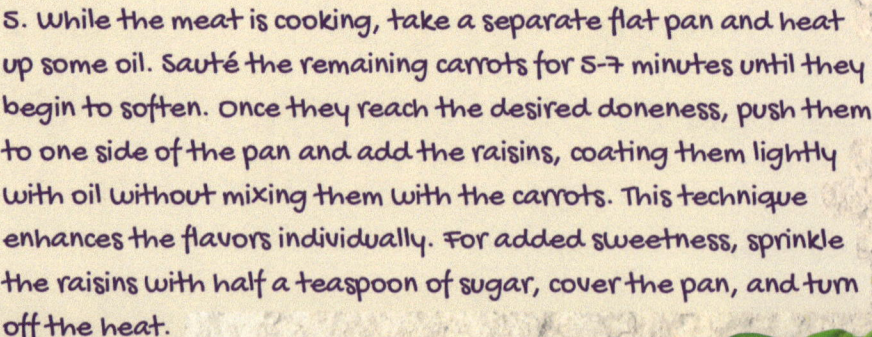

Continue:

6. After the rice has soaked, discard the excess water. Using a skimming spatula, carefully add the rice to the pot with the meat mixture, ensuring the layers remain separate. The golden rule is to have the rice covered with liquid to a depth of one finger width (approximately 3/4 of an inch). If your mixture looks dry, add more water. Gently glide the spatula to mix only the top layer of rice with the liquid, preserving the integrity of the meat and vegetables beneath. The key to mastering this dish lies in ensuring that the bottom layer remains undisturbed. Once everything is layered, add salt if needed, stir gently, and cover the pot tightly. As the dish begins to bubble, remove the lid and maintain high heat, gently pushing the rice from the edges toward the center, ensuring it cooks evenly and the bottom is not burning.

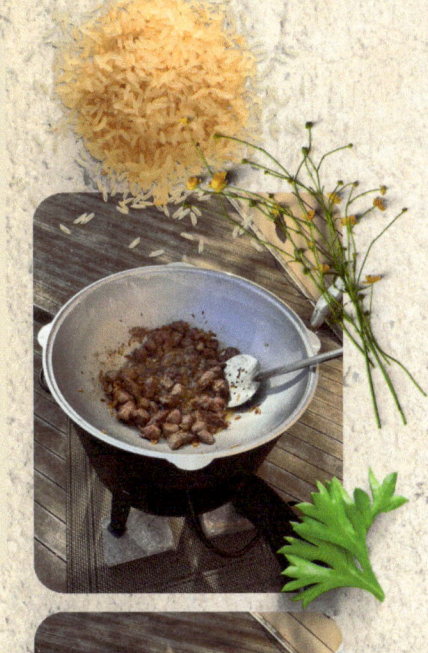

7. When you realize all the water has been absorbed, it's time to begin the steaming process known as Damla. Lower the heat to a gentle simmer. With the bottom of a wooden spatula, make several holes in the rice to allow steam to escape. If desired, sprinkle a bit more cumin on top for flavor. For an optional kick, add a whole jalapeño to steam, removing it before serving. Take a thin kitchen cloth and place it under the lid, holding it tightly while covering the pot to seal in the moisture—be careful to avoid letting any cloth hang out to prevent triggering the fire alarm. Let the rice steam for 10 minutes before turning off the heat. Allow it to rest for an additional five minutes.

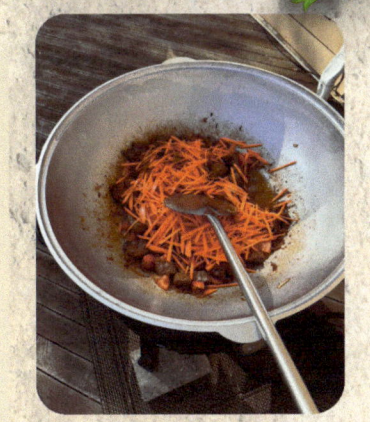

8. To serve, start layering the top portion of the rice first on a traditional serving plate, fluffing it gently with the tip of the spatula if necessary. As you approach the meat, carefully mix the succulent meat and carrots with the remaining rice. When you are ready to plate, toss the meat over the rice to enhance its fluffiness and visual appeal.

9. Serve the dish immediately, and savor the delightful flavors! Enjoy every bite of this beautifully crafted meal.

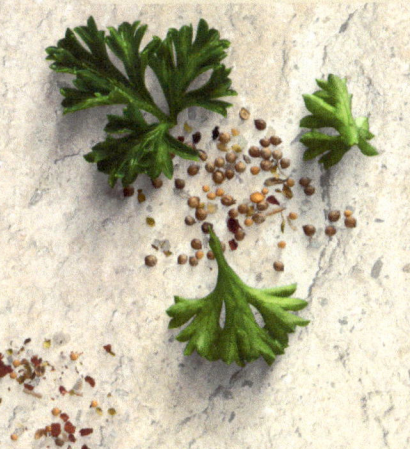

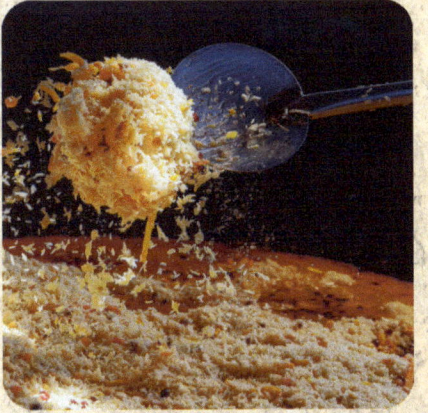

Freezing Tip: (upto 5 months)

Once you have successfully mastered step 4, it's a good idea to prepare an extra batch of the rice base. After cooling it completely, store the base in glass containers suitable for freezing. For the best results, thaw the base for about 2 hours before use, then bring it to a boil before adding the soaked rice.

REFRESHING

Persian Salad

1- Begin by thinly slicing one medium red onion and soaking the slices in cold water for 5 minutes. Squeeze out the excess water for a crisp texture.

2- Chop two firm Persian cucumbers and one large organic tomato into bite-sized pieces.

3- Add the juice of one fresh lemon, a pinch of salt, and a seeded, thinly sliced jalapeño for heat.

4- Toss all the ingredients together in a bowl. Serve this refreshing salad alongside rice for a light meal or as a flavorful side dish. Enjoy!

Neon Chutney Recipe:

- Half a bunch of fresh cilantro, chopped
- 1 teaspoon minced garlic
- 2 cups plain whole milk organic yogurt
- Salt, to taste
- Optional: 1 jalapeño, chopped (for added heat)

1. In a small blender, combine cilantro, garlic, yogurt, and salt. Add the jalapeño if you prefer a spicy kick.

2. Blend until smooth and creamy, scraping down the sides as needed.

3. Taste and adjust seasoning. For a thinner consistency, add a splash of water or more yogurt.

4. Serve immediately or store in an airtight container in the fridge for up to three days. Enjoy with Uzbek rice or as a dip!

Sweet & Sour Green Chutney

Ingredients:

1 bunch of organic cilantro: Thoroughly washed.

1 jalapeño pepper: Seeded and chopped (adjust for spice level).

½ cup filtered water

½ cup high-quality white vinegar

Salt: To taste.

½ cup golden raisins

½ cup walnuts

Instructions:

1. Blend: Combine the cilantro, jalapeño, water, vinegar, salt, raisins, and walnuts in a blender until smooth. Adjust the consistency with more water if needed.

2. Taste: Adjust salt or vinegar to achieve your desired balance of sweetness and tang.

3. Store: Transfer to an airtight container and refrigerate for up to three weeks.

This vibrant chutney is perfect for adding flavor to a variety of dishes!

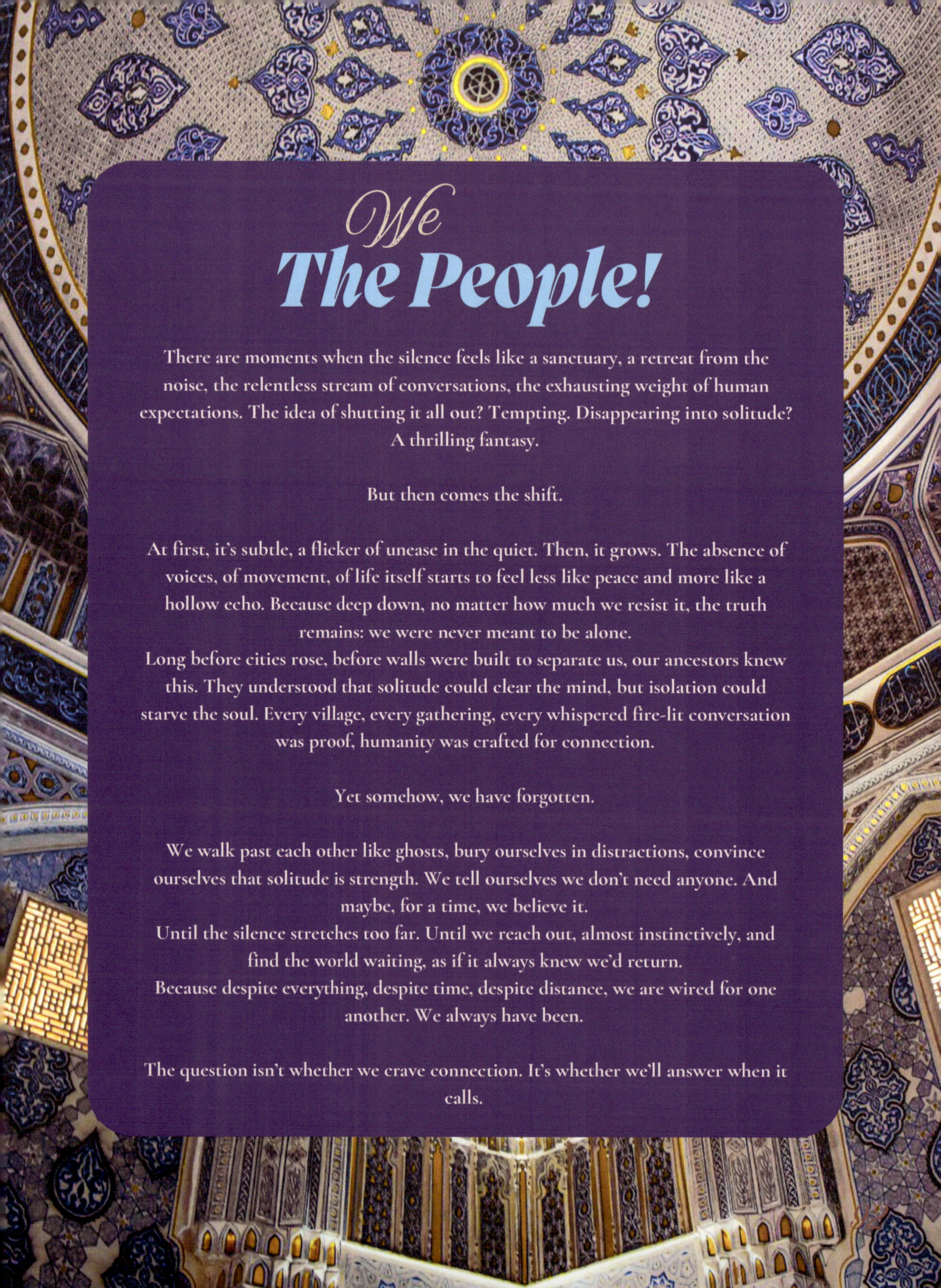

We
The People!

There are moments when the silence feels like a sanctuary, a retreat from the noise, the relentless stream of conversations, the exhausting weight of human expectations. The idea of shutting it all out? Tempting. Disappearing into solitude? A thrilling fantasy.

But then comes the shift.

At first, it's subtle, a flicker of unease in the quiet. Then, it grows. The absence of voices, of movement, of life itself starts to feel less like peace and more like a hollow echo. Because deep down, no matter how much we resist it, the truth remains: we were never meant to be alone.

Long before cities rose, before walls were built to separate us, our ancestors knew this. They understood that solitude could clear the mind, but isolation could starve the soul. Every village, every gathering, every whispered fire-lit conversation was proof, humanity was crafted for connection.

Yet somehow, we have forgotten.

We walk past each other like ghosts, bury ourselves in distractions, convince ourselves that solitude is strength. We tell ourselves we don't need anyone. And maybe, for a time, we believe it.

Until the silence stretches too far. Until we reach out, almost instinctively, and find the world waiting, as if it always knew we'd return.

Because despite everything, despite time, despite distance, we are wired for one another. We always have been.

The question isn't whether we crave connection. It's whether we'll answer when it calls.

The Final Runway

They came dressed in black - not mourning black, but couture black. The kind of black that whispers exclusive collection. Heels sharp enough to wound, handbags swinging like trophies, sunglasses still perched though the sun had long set. It was less a farewell and more a runway, a scene so rehearsed it felt like the finale of a fashion house's dream-but the grief never made it to the stage.

The woman we gathered for had been luminous, generous, unforgettable. Yet her send-off felt curated, as if sorrow itself had been styled by a consultant. Black, the color that absorbs all light, seemed to mirror the room - elegant on the surface, hollow underneath.

I thought of my grandfather's funeral decades ago. No one cared about appearances. Shirts were wrinkled, eyes swollen, voices cracked. People clung to each other, unashamed of their tears. Grief was messy, but it was real. It bound us together in a way that felt unshakable.

Now, funerals feel different. The tears are rationed, the embraces polite, the sorrow muted. Perhaps it's what happens when a world is asked to endure too much - when loss becomes background noise, when headlines bruise the spirit daily. The heart, overwhelmed, chooses silence.

But silence is dangerous. Because when grief is muted, so is joy. When sorrow is staged, so is love. And a community that forgets how to mourn forgets how to live.

Maybe that's why the handbags gleam brighter, the shoes click louder, the black grows glossier. It's easier to polish the surface than to face the fracture underneath. Easier to look immaculate than to admit we are breaking.

Yet the soul is not fooled. It waits. It waits for the crack in the performance, for the moment when the mask slips, for the flood that no designer fabric can hold back. Because numbness is not permanent - it is only borrowed time. And when the dam bursts, it will not ask permission.

So let the runway of grief continue if it must. But know this: the soul will have the last word.

Kitchrey: The Soul's Embrace

The Dance of Flavor: Ingredients for 4 servings

- Mung beans 1 cup (split or whole, rinsed)
- Sushi rice 3/4 cup, rinsed
- Water 6 cups total, divided
- Onion 1 large, finely chopped
- Garlic 4 cloves, minced, divided
- Ginger 1 tablespoon fresh, minced or grated
- Garam masala 1 teaspoon
- Turmeric 1 teaspoon
- Ground cumin 1 teaspoon, divided
- Black pepper 1/2 teaspoon
- Salt 1 1/2 teaspoons, plus more to taste
- Tomato paste 1 tablespoon (or 2 tablespoons fresh tomato purée)
- Vegetable bouillon paste or stock 1 tablespoon (or 1 cup vegetable stock instead of part of the water)
- Neutral oil 2 tablespoons (ghee if not vegan)
- Optional finishing oil 2 tablespoons neutral oil infused with 2 cloves caramelized garlic and a pinch of cayenne
- Optional garnishes dried mint, chopped cilantro, plain yogurt or labneh, toasted nuts or seeds

Instructions:

1. Sauté aromatics
   - Heat 2 tablespoons oil over medium heat. Add the chopped onion and a pinch of salt. Cook, stirring occasionally, until deeply golden and soft, 12 to 15 minutes. This caramelization adds richness; don't rush it.
   - Add 2 cloves minced garlic and the ginger; cook 30 to 45 seconds until fragrant.
2. Bloom the spices and tomato
   - Lower the heat. Add 1 teaspoon garam masala, 1 teaspoon turmeric, 1/2 teaspoon ground cumin, 1/2 teaspoon black pepper. Stir for 20 to 30 seconds until fragrant.
   - Stir in 1 tablespoon tomato paste and cook 1 minute to brown it slightly.
3. Add beans and simmer
   - Add the rinsed mung beans and 3 cups water. Bring to a gentle simmer, cover, and cook 15 to 20 minutes until the beans begin to soften but are not fully done. Check once and add water if it looks dry.

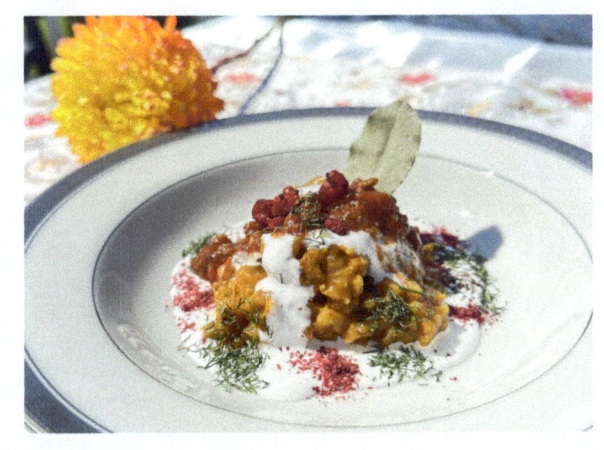

For an extra dose of nourishing goodness, swap potatoes for cubed turnips, perfect for a light cold or when craving a low-carb, plant-based option.

4- Add rice and finish cooking:

Add the rinsed sushi rice, the remaining 3 cups water, 1 tablespoon bouillon paste or 1 cup stock, and the remaining 1/2 teaspoon ground cumin and 1/2 teaspoon salt. Stir once, bring to a low simmer, cover, and cook 20 to 25 minutes until rice and beans are tender and the texture is porridge-like. Stir once or twice during this stage to prevent sticking.

5- Rest and season:

Turn off heat, keep lid on, and let the pot rest 10 minutes. Taste and adjust salt, pepper, or spice. If it's too thick, loosen with a splash of hot water.

A Bowl Made Beautiful

Stir gently to combine. Drizzle with optional hot garlic oil, sprinkle with dried mint or dill, and serve with dollops of labneh (mixed with water, salt, and minced garlic) or yogurt, accompanied by the potato qorma or meat sauce on the side.

The Vegan Potato Qorma

- Onion 1 medium, chopped
- Garlic 1 clove, minced
- Garam masala 1/2 teaspoon
- Turmeric 1/2 teaspoon
- Salt and black pepper 1/2 teaspoon each
- Tomatoes 2 medium, diced
- Potatoes 2 medium, peeled and cubed
- Water 1 to 1 1/2 cups
- Ground cumin pinch to finish

Intructions:

Caramelize onion in 1 tablespoon oil until golden. Add garlic and spices, stir 30 seconds. Add tomatoes, cook 3 to 4 minutes. Add potatoes and water, simmer covered 15 to 20 minutes until potatoes are soft. Finish with a pinch of cumin and salt to taste.

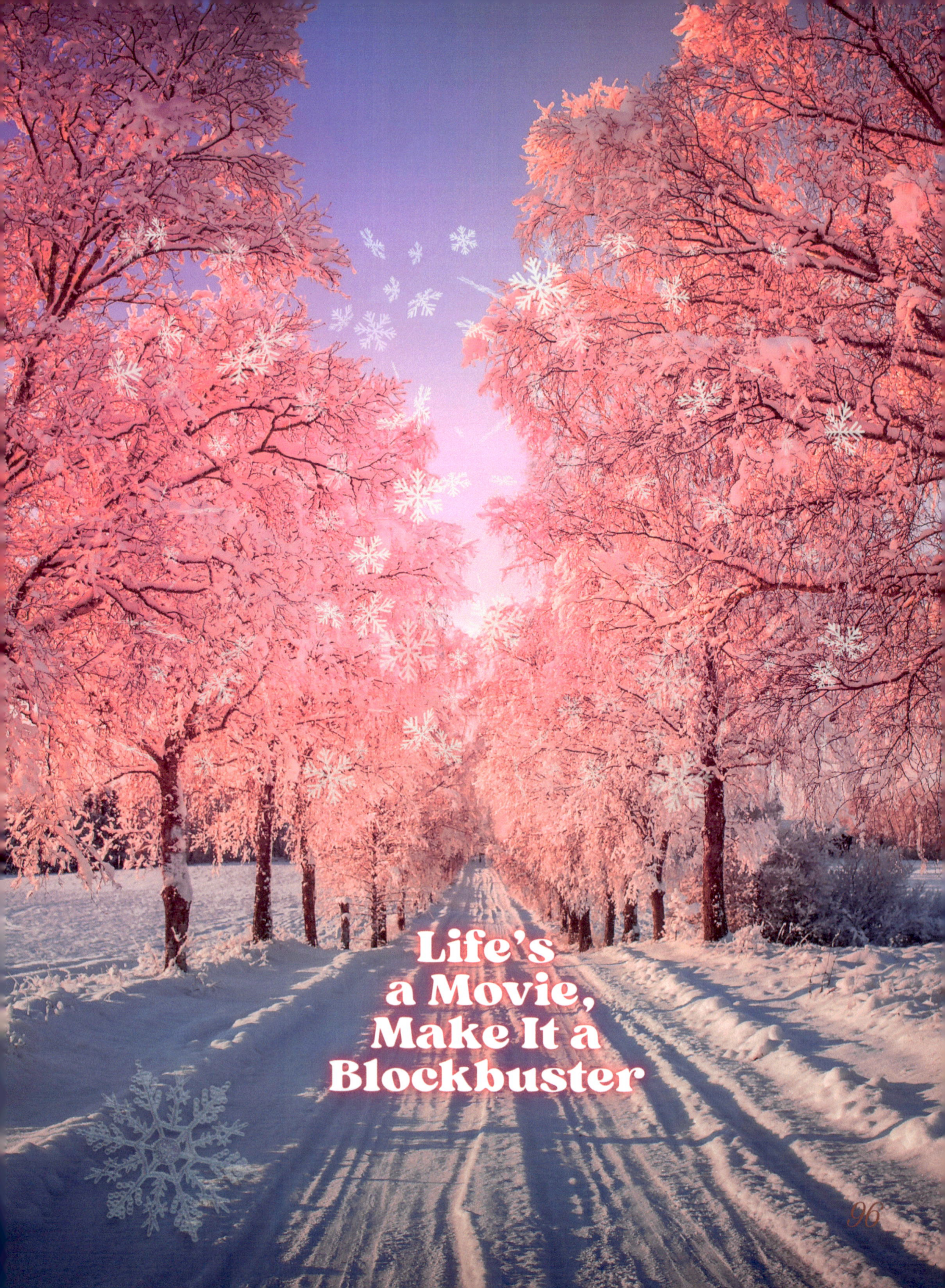

Life's a Movie, Make It a Blockbuster

A few years ago a dark, oppressive ghost gripped me, pressing the days so flat that gratitude slid away like cold butter from a plate. Small things swelled into unbearable weights; sounds made my spine tighten; I moved through rooms hollowed out, as if the part of me that knew how to want had been carved away. At night I counted the stairs to stay present; each landing a ragged, private prayer that something inside would hold.

The world's speed widened that hollow. Faces blurred into notifications; obligations ate hours I might have spent becoming myself; my edges softened until I could no longer tell which choices were truly mine. The truth landed like a slow bruise. I stopped pretending I could shoulder everything for everyone.

So I stepped back. I put devices in another room, let silence grow long enough to hear my own pulse, and learned the strange relief of being unreachable. Saying no felt like learning a new language; reclaiming small hours felt like surfacing for breath. The change was patient, fierce, and aching, quiet refusals that reshaped my days.

Cooking became the place I practiced coming home. The scrape of a spoon on a pot steadied me; heat taught me how to hold intensity without splintering; slow tending taught me to notice the small things that add up. Each recipe became a lesson in attention; each meal a proof I could choose presence over distraction. I kept phones in the other room so pings could not hollow my head, and conversations lengthened, appetite returned for life not just comfort, and my hands relearned how to stitch steadiness into the day.

Once, in a corner of a sunlit flower shop, I met an old woman who changed everything I thought courage looked like. Years earlier, after her husband died, a neighbor who had been unusually close began bringing bread and lingering near the widow's door. Rumors swelled; people braced for fury. The widow felt pulled two ways: one impulse wanted to let the betrayal define her; another, thinner and quieter, pulled her back. Months before the husband's final illness, she'd slipped a scrap of paper into a cookbook and written one line for the future version of herself: *I will not let my life be borrowed*. On the day the warm loaf arrived her hand brushed that scrap as she opened the door-an anchor in a sudden current. She took the bread, set it on the small table in her kitchen, and invited the neighbor in. She did not perform forgiveness; she named her grief and set her boundary in plain, steady sentences. The neighbor did not deny what had been; the widow's steadiness simply unmoored shame from power. The surprise the woman told me was not a spectacle but a simple, explosive truth: she claimed the shape of her days not by grand absolution but by refusing to let betrayal write her life.

When I visited her shop that spring, the place hummed with small bright things—bunches of ranunculus, a boy buying a bundle to apologize, a neighbor picking up flowers for a new baby. The woman moved between stems with the calm of someone who has practiced keeping her hands busy on purpose. She showed me the recipe card with the folded scrap taped to the back and laughed softly: she'd kept that line through winters and weddings and mornings she could not breathe. The shop felt like a living proof: steady tending makes a life that holds.

Healing came to me the same way, through repeated returns. A shared bowl that let laughter leak back; a clear morning when the sky read as possibility; the slow rebuilding of appetite for life rather than its comforts. In my kitchen, I practiced the discipline of attention-keeping screens away, stirring until the sauce and the tightness in my chest both loosened, choosing again and again what fills me instead of what drains me. I did not simply slip away from the shadow; I rebuilt around presence, fidelity to small acts, and the courage to refuse what is hollow.

I found cooking-fresh air and a map; I found cooking-what's your way out?

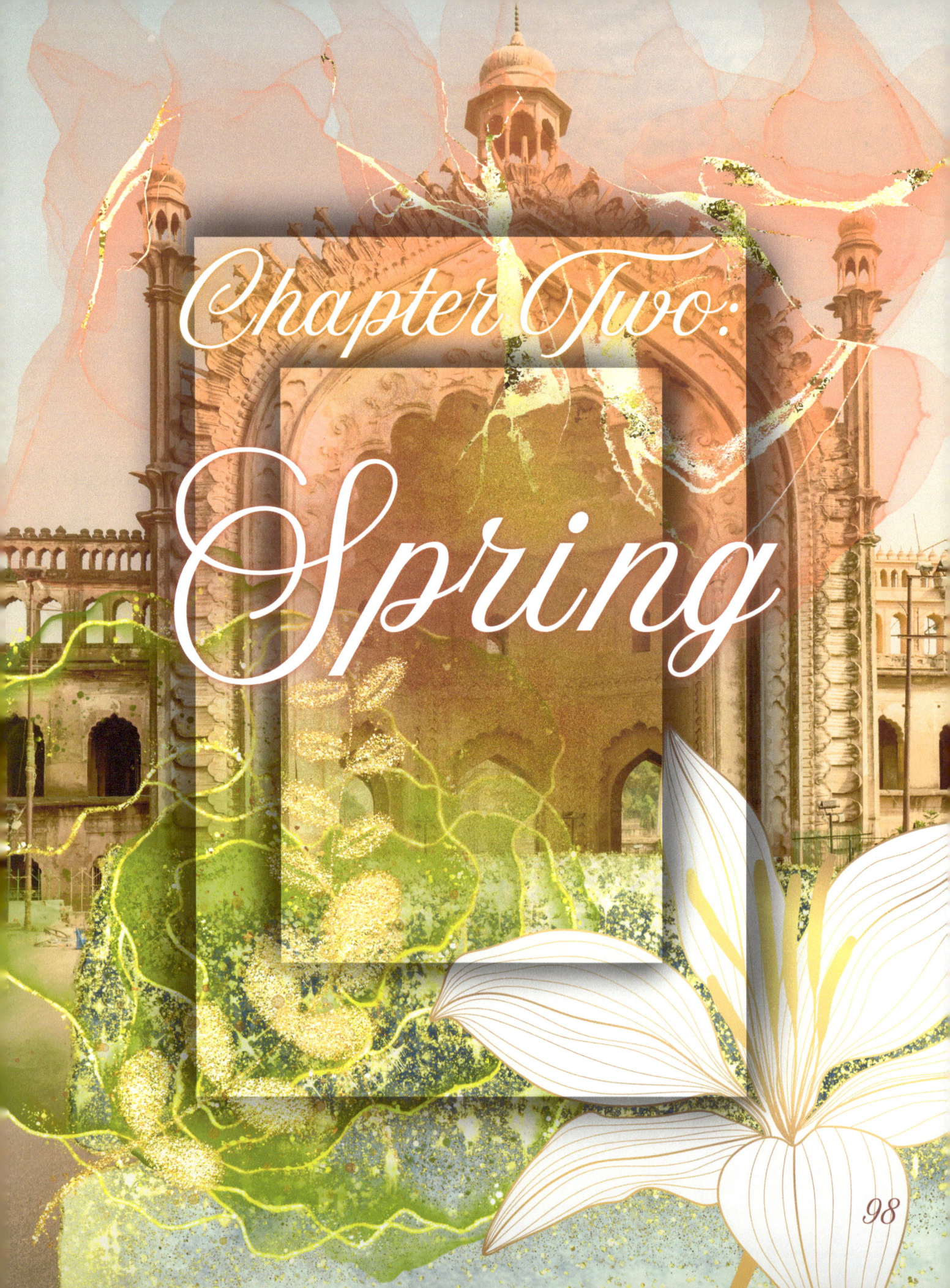

Chapter Two:
Spring

Violent in Its Beauty

Spring is not gentle. It is violent in its beauty - buds splitting open, rivers breaking free, light flooding places that forgot it existed. And you are invited to claim that same beauty, in your own way, in your own time.

This is not a season of pastel politeness. It is a season of rupture. Roots tear through soil, branches stretch until they ache, and the world remakes itself in colors so bold they sting the eyes. Petals don't ask permission before they burst; rivers don't apologize as they overflow their banks. And perhaps you, too, can allow yourself to expand, without apology.

The new you is not a quiet unveiling. You may arrive like a drumbeat after silence, like green cracking concrete, like a body remembering its own voltage. Not rushed, not forced - simply inevitable. You don't need to wait for approval, you don't need to shrink to fit. You are the surge and the bloom, the tide and the blaze of color.

This season is not about tiptoeing into change. It is about allowing yourself to open, to radiate, to step into a self that feels more alive, more undeniable. Every breath can be sharper, every choice more deliberate, every step a quiet declaration that you are moving beyond the muted life you once endured.

Spring proves that rebirth is not delicate - it is ferocious. Yet ferocity doesn't have to mean harm; it can mean courage, vibrancy, unapologetic presence. The earth cracks, the air thickens with pollen and promise, the sky dares you to look up and believe again. And so does this becoming. Not soft, not subtle - but vivid, expansive, unstoppable in its own rhythm.

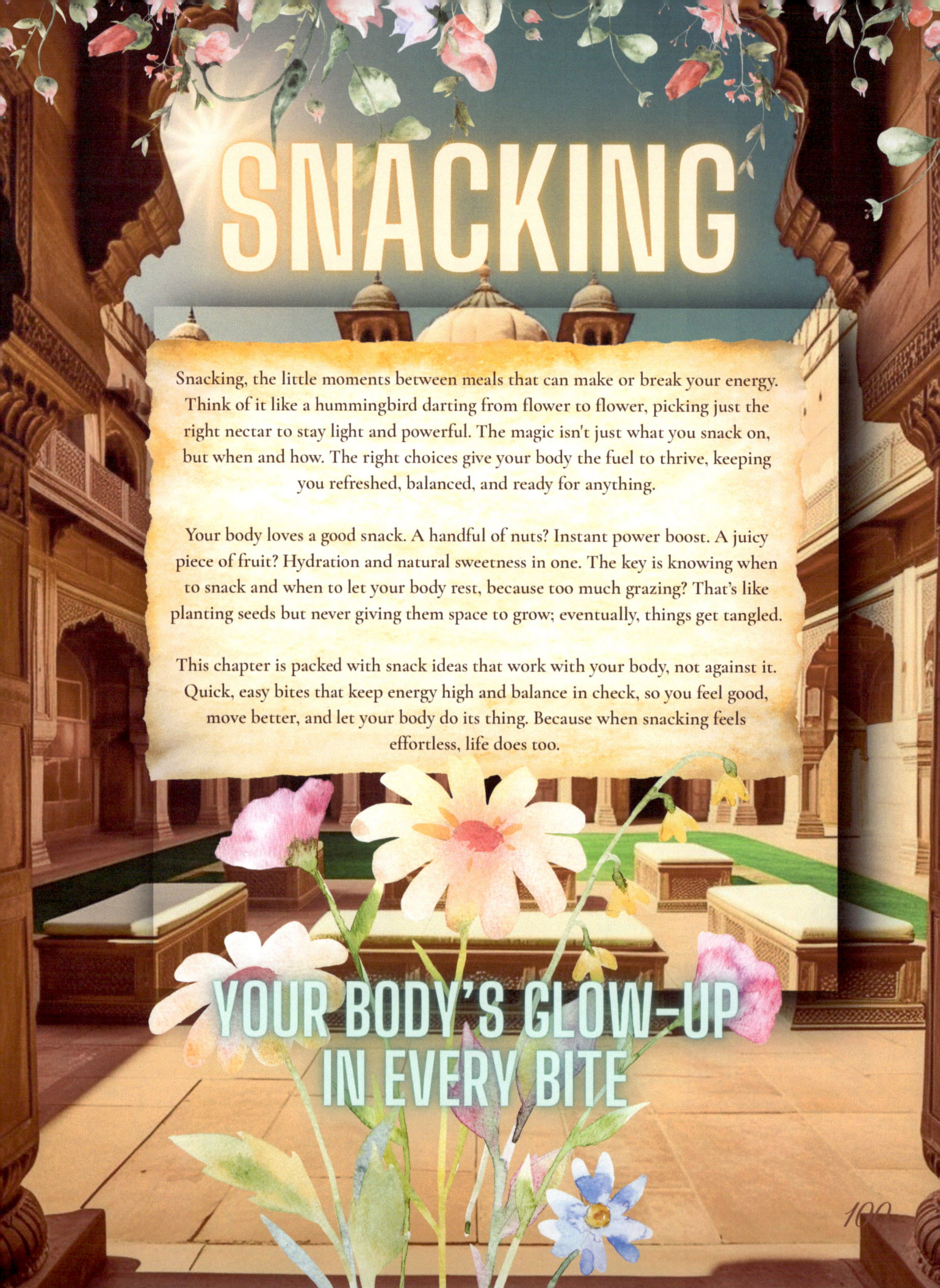

SNACKING

Snacking, the little moments between meals that can make or break your energy. Think of it like a hummingbird darting from flower to flower, picking just the right nectar to stay light and powerful. The magic isn't just what you snack on, but when and how. The right choices give your body the fuel to thrive, keeping you refreshed, balanced, and ready for anything.

Your body loves a good snack. A handful of nuts? Instant power boost. A juicy piece of fruit? Hydration and natural sweetness in one. The key is knowing when to snack and when to let your body rest, because too much grazing? That's like planting seeds but never giving them space to grow; eventually, things get tangled.

This chapter is packed with snack ideas that work with your body, not against it. Quick, easy bites that keep energy high and balance in check, so you feel good, move better, and let your body do its thing. Because when snacking feels effortless, life does too.

YOUR BODY'S GLOW-UP IN EVERY BITE

Snack Smarter in a Synthetic World

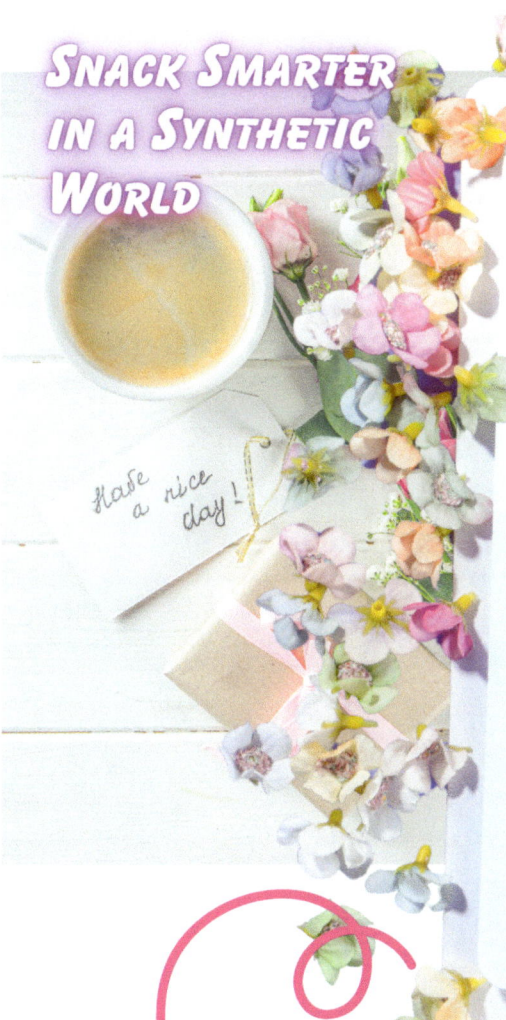

Have a nice day!

In the great chemical jungle we call modern life, many of us are swimming in a sea of synthetic stuff our bodies don't even recognize! These sneaky compounds can really shake up our bodily functions, which isn't great news for our health. Take endocrine disruptors like Bisphenol A (BPA), for example, they're like the uninvited guests that mess with our metabolism and throw our hormonal balance into chaos. This is a major plot twist for women over 40, who are already juggling hormonal fireworks and trying to keep weight in check. What a wild ride!

BPA is commonly found in a myriad of everyday products, including nonstick cookware, plastic containers, food and beverage packaging, toys, cosmetics, detergents, and pesticides. Its widespread use raises serious concerns about long-term exposure and accumulation in our bodies.

Continue

Snack Timing That Supports Weight & Hormonal Balance

The effects of these chemicals can extend beyond individual health, as they also contribute to broader environmental pollution, affecting air and soil quality.

The reality of chemical exposure is alarming and warrants serious reflection. It's crucial that we become more aware of how our snacks are prepared and stored, and take actionable steps to minimize exposure to harmful substances. By opting for safer materials, such as glass, stainless steel, or ceramic, and being mindful of the food packaging we choose, we can make a significant difference in our health and the environment.

Snack timing isn't just about curbing cravings, it's about syncing with your body's natural energy and metabolism:

- Mid-morning (10–11 a.m.): Ideal for keeping blood sugar stable and avoiding energy dips. Pair fruit with nuts or seeds.
- Mid-afternoon (3–4 p.m.): Supports focus and mood. Try fiber-rich snacks like veggie sticks with hummus or a savory chia bowl.
- Avoid late-night snacking (after 8 p.m.): The body's digestion slows down, increasing fat storage and disrupting sleep.

Simple shifts in when and how you snack can lead to meaningful changes, not just in how you feel, but in how your body thrives.

Mango:

Can anything in Mother Nature's pantry compete with the lip-smacking taste and luscious texture of a mango? Its juicy, satisfying flesh gives avocados a run for their money! This delightful gem is easily one of my top two fruit crushes. Packed with skin-saving vitamins C and A plus a boatload of antioxidants, it's like a fruity superhero fighting inflammation and boosting that glow-up!

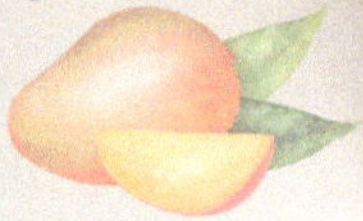

Pomegranate:

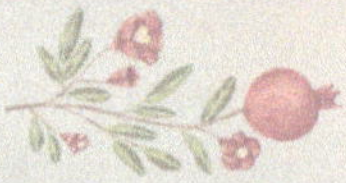

Pomegranate is the star of fruits, packing a health punch like no other! I'm head over heels for this juicy gem, I could munch on it from dawn till dusk! It's a champion at squashing inflammation, kicking cancer risks to the curb, keeping your ticker happy, powering up your immune defenses, calming high blood pressure, and giving your brain a high-five! Plus, it's loaded with fiber, vitamin C, and vitamin K, talk about a fruity triple threat!

Celery:

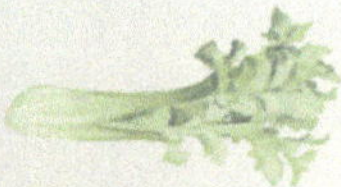

- Hydration - check

- Vitamin K, magnesium, calcium - check

- Bone health - check

- Anti-inflammatory, antioxidant - check

- Boost immune system - check

- Gut health - check

- Healthy pH balance - check

- Stress be gone - check

- Snack attack approved - double-check!

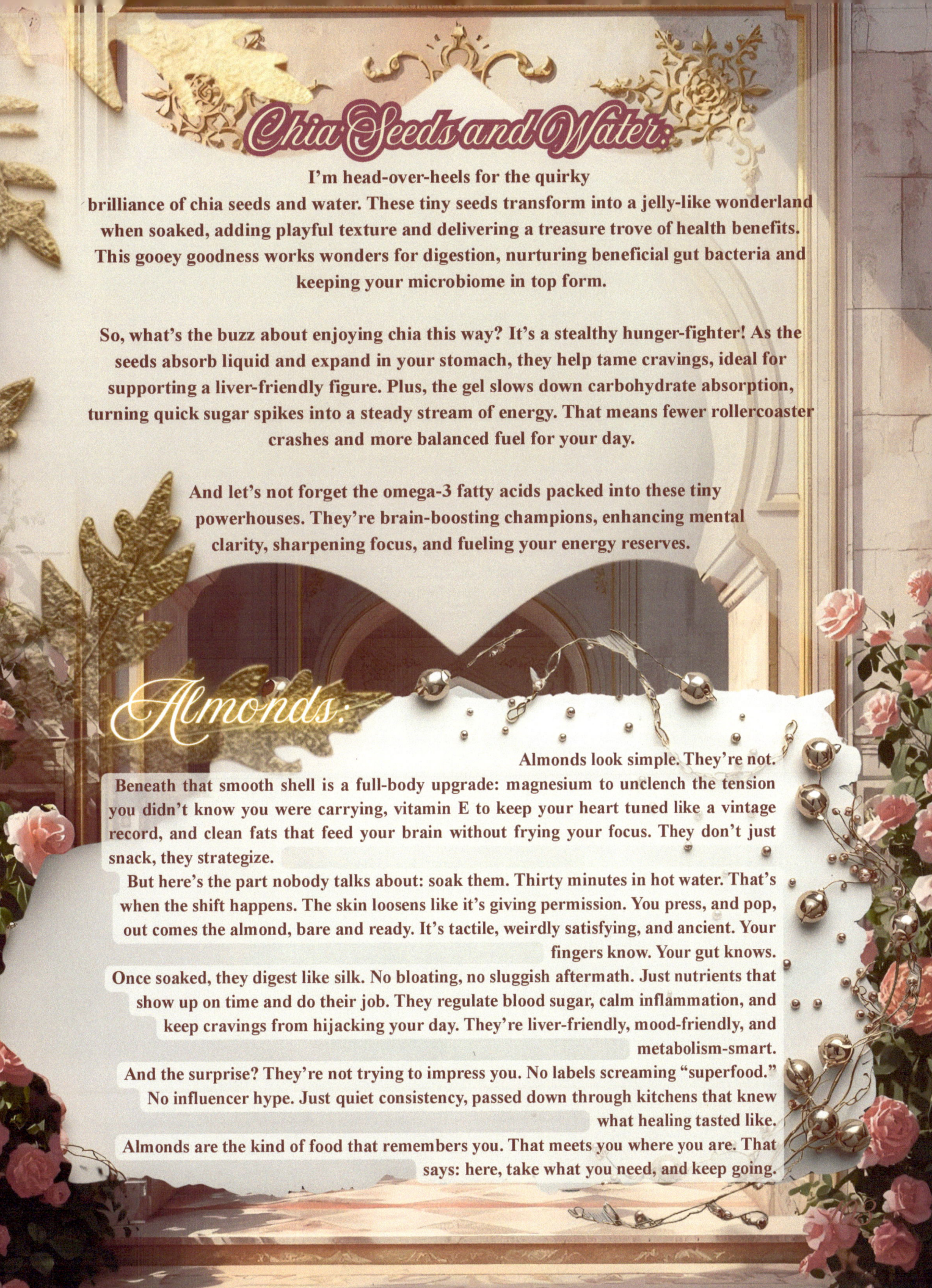

Chia Seeds and Water:

I'm head-over-heels for the quirky
brilliance of chia seeds and water. These tiny seeds transform into a jelly-like wonderland
when soaked, adding playful texture and delivering a treasure trove of health benefits.
This gooey goodness works wonders for digestion, nurturing beneficial gut bacteria and
keeping your microbiome in top form.

So, what's the buzz about enjoying chia this way? It's a stealthy hunger-fighter! As the
seeds absorb liquid and expand in your stomach, they help tame cravings, ideal for
supporting a liver-friendly figure. Plus, the gel slows down carbohydrate absorption,
turning quick sugar spikes into a steady stream of energy. That means fewer rollercoaster
crashes and more balanced fuel for your day.

And let's not forget the omega-3 fatty acids packed into these tiny
powerhouses. They're brain-boosting champions, enhancing mental
clarity, sharpening focus, and fueling your energy reserves.

Almonds:

Almonds look simple. They're not.
Beneath that smooth shell is a full-body upgrade: magnesium to unclench the tension
you didn't know you were carrying, vitamin E to keep your heart tuned like a vintage
record, and clean fats that feed your brain without frying your focus. They don't just
snack, they strategize.

But here's the part nobody talks about: soak them. Thirty minutes in hot water. That's
when the shift happens. The skin loosens like it's giving permission. You press, and pop,
out comes the almond, bare and ready. It's tactile, weirdly satisfying, and ancient. Your
fingers know. Your gut knows.
Once soaked, they digest like silk. No bloating, no sluggish aftermath. Just nutrients that
show up on time and do their job. They regulate blood sugar, calm inflammation, and
keep cravings from hijacking your day. They're liver-friendly, mood-friendly, and
metabolism-smart.
And the surprise? They're not trying to impress you. No labels screaming "superfood."
No influencer hype. Just quiet consistency, passed down through kitchens that knew
what healing tasted like.
Almonds are the kind of food that remembers you. That meets you where you are. That
says: here, take what you need, and keep going.

The Root Touch-Up That Changed Everything

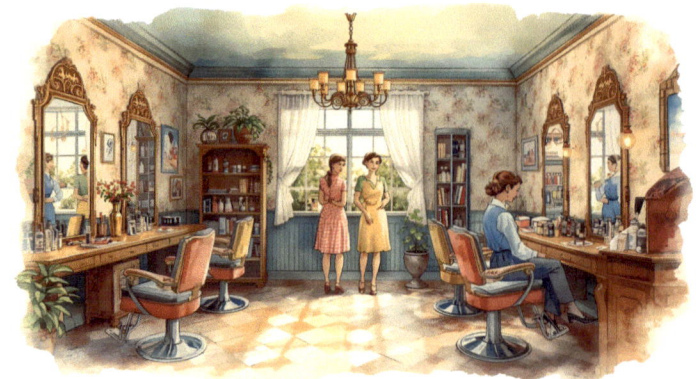

She came for color. She left with clarity

Back when I owned my salon, a woman came in for a simple trim, but what unraveled in the chair was anything but simple. She'd just clawed her way out of a brutal divorce, only to fall into the arms of someone new. He was charming, attentive, and (according to her) "a fresh start." But something felt off. Her energy was low, her skin dull, her digestion a mess. She joked that he was "draining her," and I remember thinking: maybe he was.

Four weeks later, she was back in my chair for her root touch-up. Same smile, but something had shifted. She leaned in and said, "You're not going to believe this, I have parasites." Real ones. Her doctor had found them in her gut. Tiny invaders feeding off her from the inside out. The irony wasn't lost on either of us. She'd welcomed a man who mirrored the very thing happening in her body: something that looked harmless but stole her vitality.
Instead of prescriptions, she opted for a holistic approach. Oil of oregano became her weapon of choice; potent, ancient, and wildly effective. She paired it with clove, wormwood, and a gut-friendly diet that starved the invaders and rebuilt her strength. Slowly, her body cleared.

Her mind followed.
And then came the deeper release.
She let go of the man. She realized he wasn't love; he was a pattern. A familiar kind of erosion. And with that clarity came another: her ex-husband, the mental parasite she'd been carrying long after the papers were signed. His voice, his criticism, his shadow. Her body had been bracing for impact long after the blows had stopped.

So she began the real work. Breathwork. Journaling. Long walks without her phone. She stopped rehearsing old arguments in her head. She stopped letting his ghost shape her choices.
And slowly, the picture changed.

Her face softened. Her posture opened. Her laughter came quicker, stayed longer. It was like watching a painting restore itself, layers of tension lifted, color returned to places that had gone gray. She didn't just leave the new guy. She reclaimed the room he'd taken up. She didn't just forget the ex. She rewrote the space where his voice used to echo.
Two parasites. One physical, one emotional. Both gone.
Healing isn't always pretty. But when it's real, it's complete.

BYE-BYE PARASITE SMOOTHIE

A Gut-Loving Blend with Attitude

Caution: Oil of oregano is powerful, start small, especially if you're new to it. Not recommended during pregnancy or for children. Always check with your body (and your practitioner) before diving in.

This isn't your average green drink. It's a sassy little blend designed to kick out the freeloaders, whether they're in your belly or your life. It's anti-parasitic, anti-inflammatory, and pro-boundaries. Plus, it tastes like a tropical vacation with a side of "I deserve better."

Ingredients:

1 cup coconut water (hydrating + electrolyte-rich)
½ frozen banana (for creaminess and potassium)
½ cup pineapple chunks (bromelain = parasite kryptonite)
3 drops oil of oregano (or as directed on the bottle, this stuff is bold)
Juice of ½ lime (zesty + liver-loving)
Pinch of clove or cinnamon (warm, grounding, and gut-friendly)
Optional: 1 scoop collagen or plant protein (for repair and glow)

Instructions:

Blend until smooth. Sip with intention. Imagine the parasites packing their bags. Imagine the exes doing the same. This smoothie doesn't just taste good, it clears space.

WHY IT WORKS

Pineapple: contains bromelain, an enzyme that helps break down invaders
Oil of oregano: nature's bouncer, strong, spicy, and unapologetic
Lime: supports liver detox and adds brightness
Clove/cinnamon: warm the gut and help fight off unwanted guests
Coconut water: hydrates while keeping things moving

WHEN TO USE

During a cleanse
After a breakup
When you feel bloated, foggy, or emotionally "invaded"
As a reminder that healing can taste amazing

This smoothie is a boundary in a blender. A tropical "no thanks" to anything that doesn't serve you. Drink it cold. Drink it bold. And keep going.

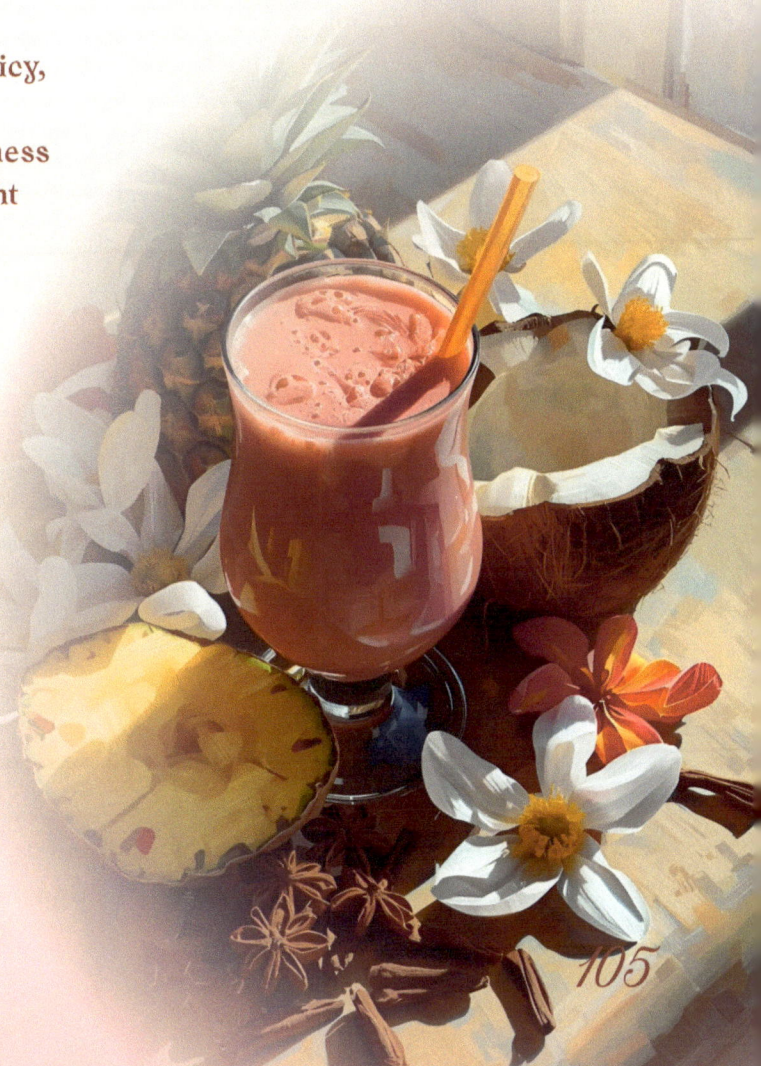

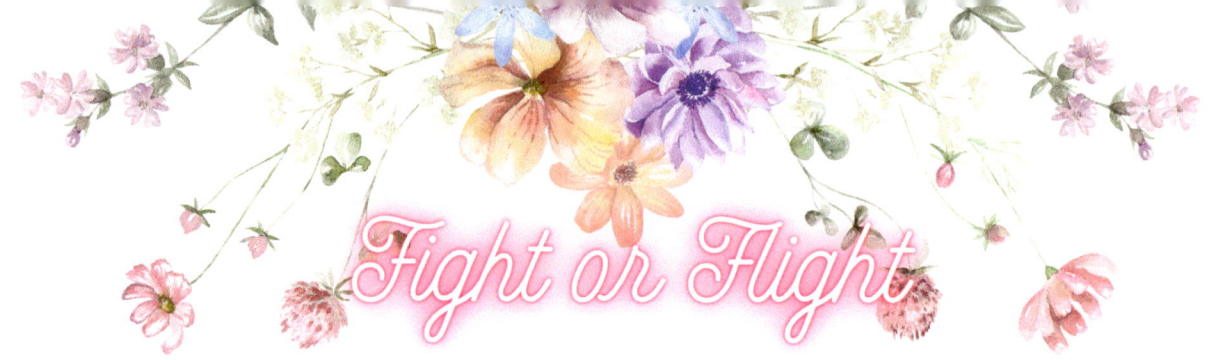

Fight or Flight

Meet the "Fight or Flight" response, your body's built-in superhero mode that kicks in when danger's lurking around the corner! This primal survival trick gears you up to either duke it out "fight" or hightail it outta there "flight." When the alarm bells ring, your autonomic nervous system, especially the sympathetic squad, jumps into action. It unleashes a thunderstorm of stress hormones, mainly adrenaline and norepinephrine, turning you into a lean, mean, survival machine!

These hormones lead to a series of rapid changes in the body: heart rate elevates to pump blood to essential muscles, blood pressure rises to keep oxygen flowing, and breathing becomes quick and shallow to supercharge oxygen intake. Pupils dilate for laser-sharp vision, and blood gets rerouted from digestion to the muscles, because
right now, surviving beats snacking.

Even your brain joins the hustle. It kicks into high gear, sharpening your focus and reaction time like a tactical commander scanning for threats and escape plans. This lightning-fast response has kept species alive for millennia, helping them dodge predators, natural disasters, and the wild curveballs nature throws.

But here's the kicker: your brain's threat-detection system doesn't need fangs or flashing sirens to go haywire, it can flip the switch from an email subject line. Chronic stress keeps the fight-or-flight circuit humming like a broken alarm, flooding the body with emergency-mode hormones even when the only predator is your calendar. Over time, this biochemical overdrive acts like silent sabotage.

Doctors call it allostatic load: a slow-burn meltdown. Cortisol stays elevated, causing sleep disruptions, insulin resistance, digestive chaos, and immune suppression. Brain fog creeps in. Energy tanks. The body starts whispering distress signals, until they become screams.
Enter the secret weapon: parasympathetic override. Not just spa-day fluff, but hardwired neurological recovery. Deep diaphragmatic breathing stimulates the vagus nerve, flipping the internal switch from "alert" to "repair." Omega-3s dampen inflammation. Adaptogens stabilize cortisol rhythms. Restorative
movement floods tissues with oxygen and reverses neural fatigue!
Translation? Strategic calm is not weakness, it's
biochemical resilience. It's the protocol elite clinicians
whisper to burnt-out executives and trauma survivors.
And it starts with reclaiming your body from false alarms.

Do Not Stress over Everything:

When stress crashes the party, your body's adrenal glands throw a cortisol bash, starring the infamous "stress hormone." While cortisol's there to get you ready for battle or a quick getaway, too much of it can turn your belly into a snack stash. And if that isn't enough, high cortisol levels might transform you into a snack-hunting machine, craving comfort foods straight from the junk food aisle.

But fear not! When your mind's chilling on a zen cloud, your body can work its wonders and heal. Stress might be a pesky guest, but when it crashes your day, take a breather. Try some deep breaths, a quick stroll, or find a cozy corner to relax. These mini vacays can be your secret tool for feeling stress-free and keeping that waistline in check.

Take your Sweet Time Chewing:

Now, let me tell you about my slow-eating buddy, a relative of mine. We're the same age and have ridden the roller coaster of life together. We've mastered the art of snail-paced munching, which might just be the secret sauce to keeping our weight in the "healthy" zone, though every family member's got their own style at the dinner table.

Chewing slow is like giving your mouth a head start in the digestive marathon. Plus, after about 20 minutes, your brain waves the "full" flag, keeping you from joining the clean plate club. This mindful munching is a superpower for portion control and dodging overeating. And the cherry on top? Savoring every single bite makes meals a deliciously epic experience!

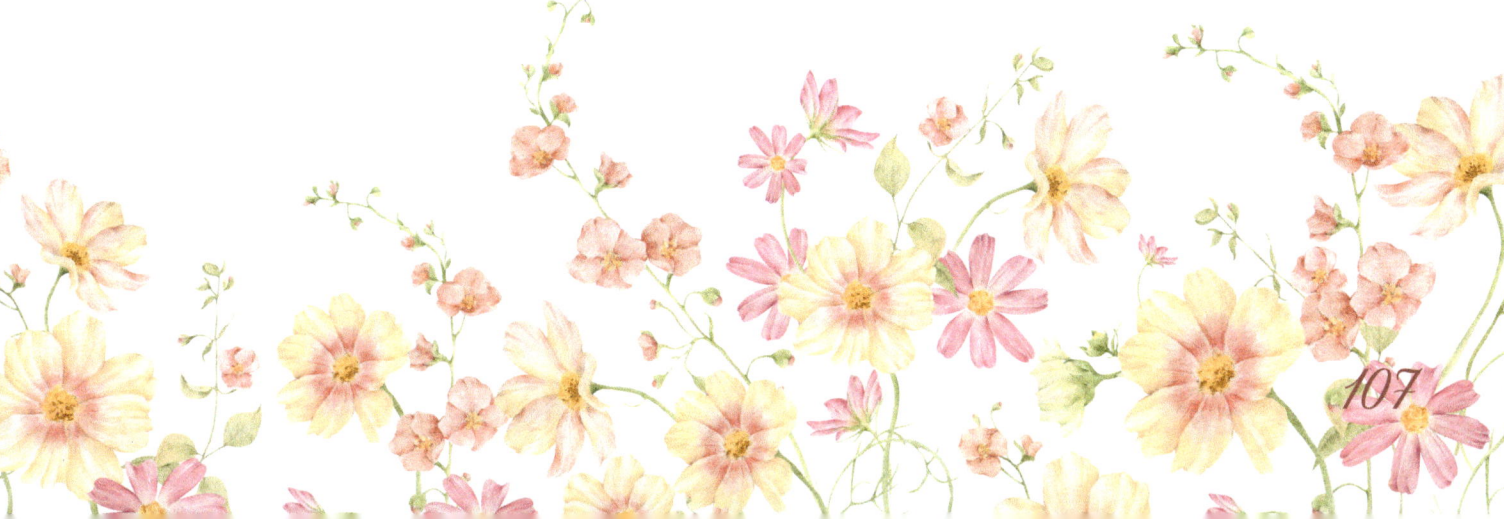

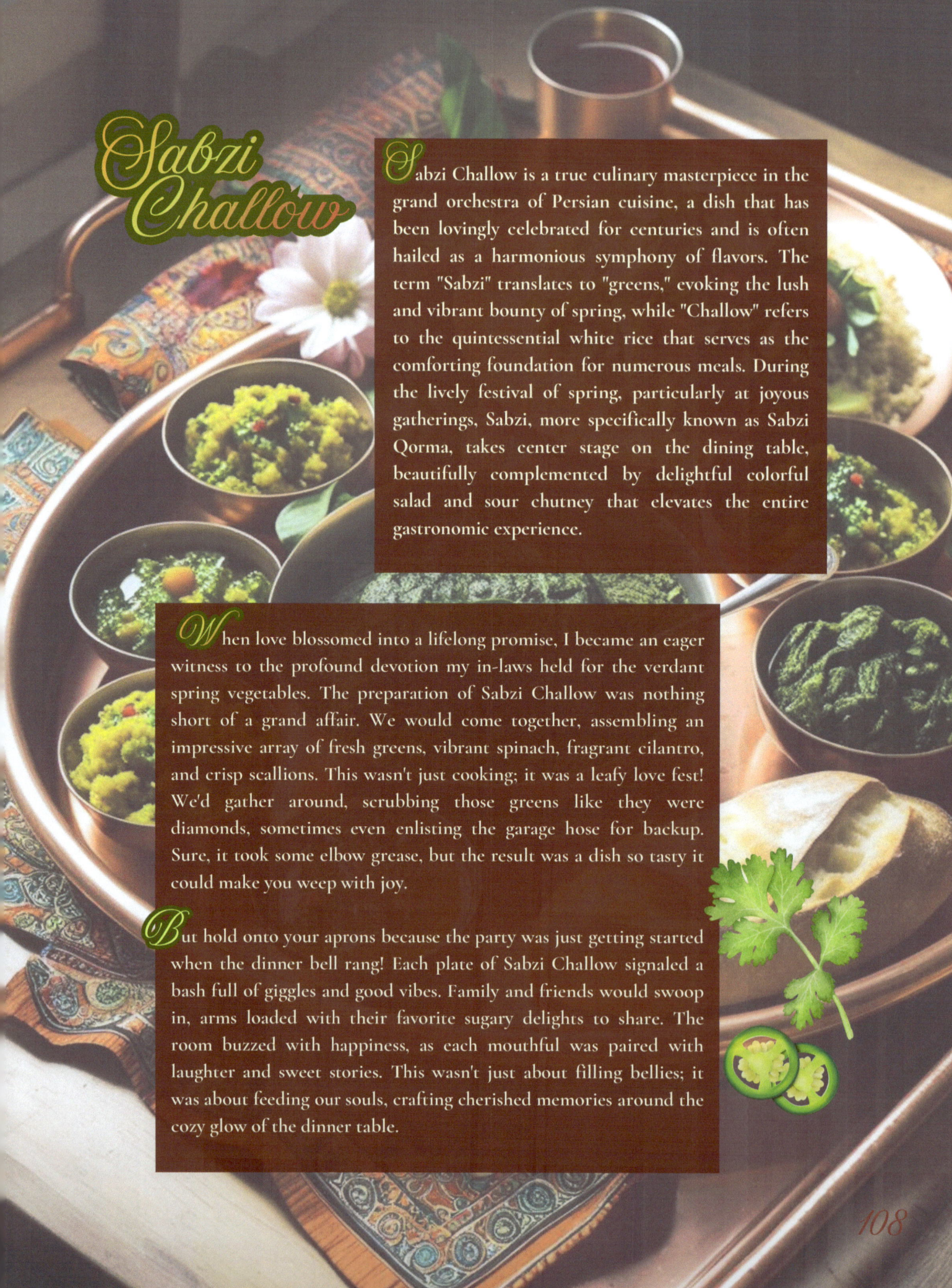

Sabzi Challow

Sabzi Challow is a true culinary masterpiece in the grand orchestra of Persian cuisine, a dish that has been lovingly celebrated for centuries and is often hailed as a harmonious symphony of flavors. The term "Sabzi" translates to "greens," evoking the lush and vibrant bounty of spring, while "Challow" refers to the quintessential white rice that serves as the comforting foundation for numerous meals. During the lively festival of spring, particularly at joyous gatherings, Sabzi, more specifically known as Sabzi Qorma, takes center stage on the dining table, beautifully complemented by delightful colorful salad and sour chutney that elevates the entire gastronomic experience.

When love blossomed into a lifelong promise, I became an eager witness to the profound devotion my in-laws held for the verdant spring vegetables. The preparation of Sabzi Challow was nothing short of a grand affair. We would come together, assembling an impressive array of fresh greens, vibrant spinach, fragrant cilantro, and crisp scallions. This wasn't just cooking; it was a leafy love fest! We'd gather around, scrubbing those greens like they were diamonds, sometimes even enlisting the garage hose for backup. Sure, it took some elbow grease, but the result was a dish so tasty it could make you weep with joy.

But hold onto your aprons because the party was just getting started when the dinner bell rang! Each plate of Sabzi Challow signaled a bash full of giggles and good vibes. Family and friends would swoop in, arms loaded with their favorite sugary delights to share. The room buzzed with happiness, as each mouthful was paired with laughter and sweet stories. This wasn't just about filling bellies; it was about feeding our souls, crafting cherished memories around the cozy glow of the dinner table.

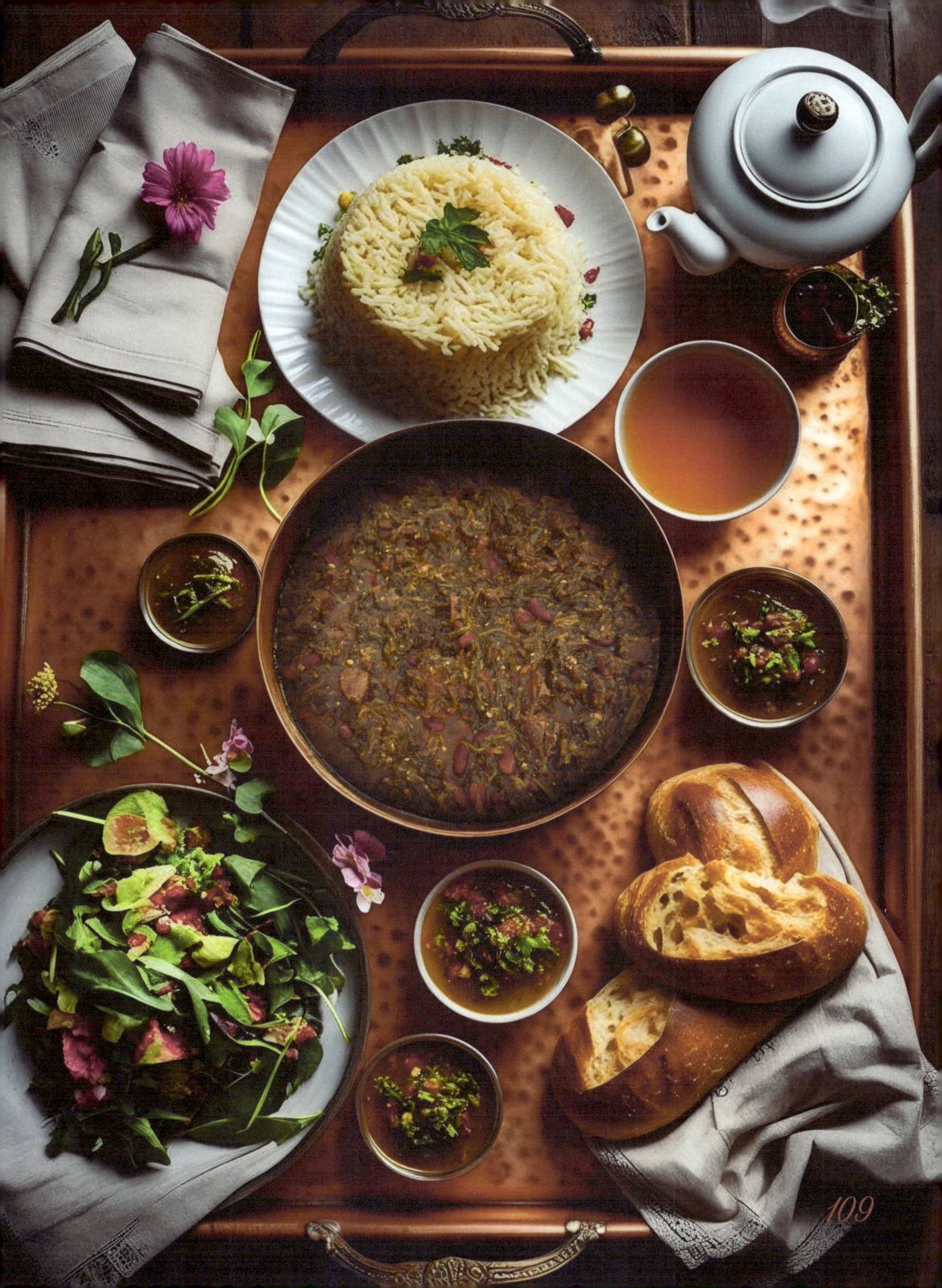

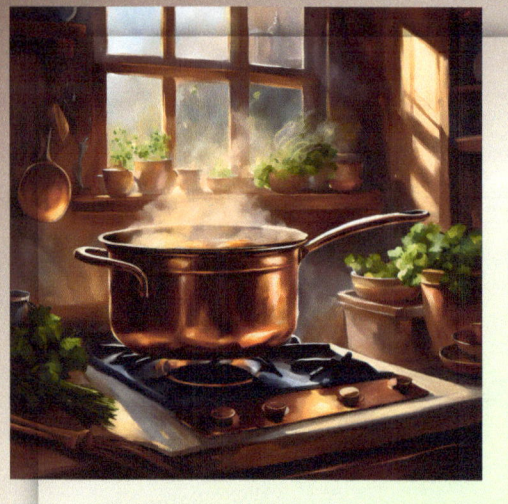

Ingredients:

- ½ cup avocado oil
- One large organic yellow onion cut into thin slices
- One tablespoon of minced garlic
- Two teaspoons of organic tomato paste
- One tablespoon turmeric
- Salt and black pepper
- One tablespoon fenugreek (optional)
- One cup of dry kidney beans (washed and soaked in hot water for an hour)
- One bunch of cilantros, washed and chopped
- ½ a cup of homemade beef gelatin (optional)
- One large bag of pre-washed baby spinach
- one bunch of dill washed and chopped
- One bunch of scallions washed and cut into small pieces
- ¼ teaspoon cayenne pepper
- Water

Instructions for Sabzi Qorma:

1. **Prepare the Pot:** Start by placing a large, deep stainless steel pot on the stove over medium heat. Allow it to heat for about one minute to ensure an even temperature.

2. **Add Oil:***Pour in avocado oil and let it heat for an additional 30 seconds. The oil should shimmer slightly, indicating it's ready for cooking.

3. **Caramelize the Onions:** Add thinly sliced onions to the hot oil. Stir occasionally, allowing them to caramelize gently for 5-7 minutes. You want the onions to become translucent and develop a golden brown color, enhancing the flavor of your dish.

4. **Beef Beauty Pageant:** Time for the beef cubes to enter into the pot! Shower them with a sprinkle of salt and a dash of freshly cracked black pepper. Crank up the heat to high and let those cubes sizzle, flipping them around until they're gorgeously bronzed on all sides. This stage is key for crafting that mouthwatering, flavor-packed stew!

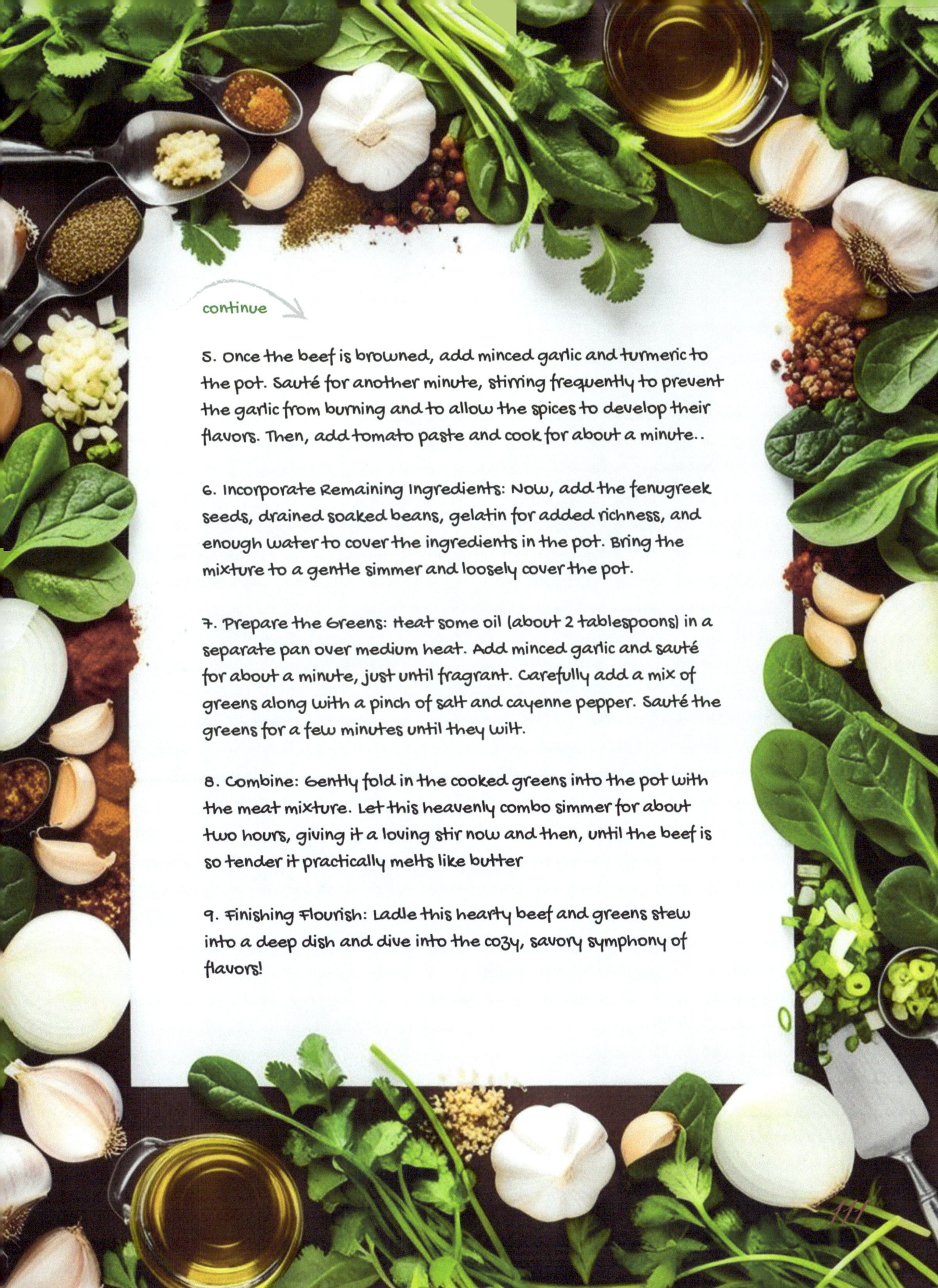

continue

5. Once the beef is browned, add minced garlic and turmeric to the pot. Sauté for another minute, stirring frequently to prevent the garlic from burning and to allow the spices to develop their flavors. Then, add tomato paste and cook for about a minute..

6. Incorporate Remaining Ingredients: Now, add the fenugreek seeds, drained soaked beans, gelatin for added richness, and enough water to cover the ingredients in the pot. Bring the mixture to a gentle simmer and loosely cover the pot.

7. Prepare the Greens: Heat some oil (about 2 tablespoons) in a separate pan over medium heat. Add minced garlic and sauté for about a minute, just until fragrant. Carefully add a mix of greens along with a pinch of salt and cayenne pepper. Sauté the greens for a few minutes until they wilt.

8. Combine: Gently fold in the cooked greens into the pot with the meat mixture. Let this heavenly combo simmer for about two hours, giving it a loving stir now and then, until the beef is so tender it practically melts like butter

9. Finishing Flourish: Ladle this hearty beef and greens stew into a deep dish and dive into the cozy, savory symphony of flavors!

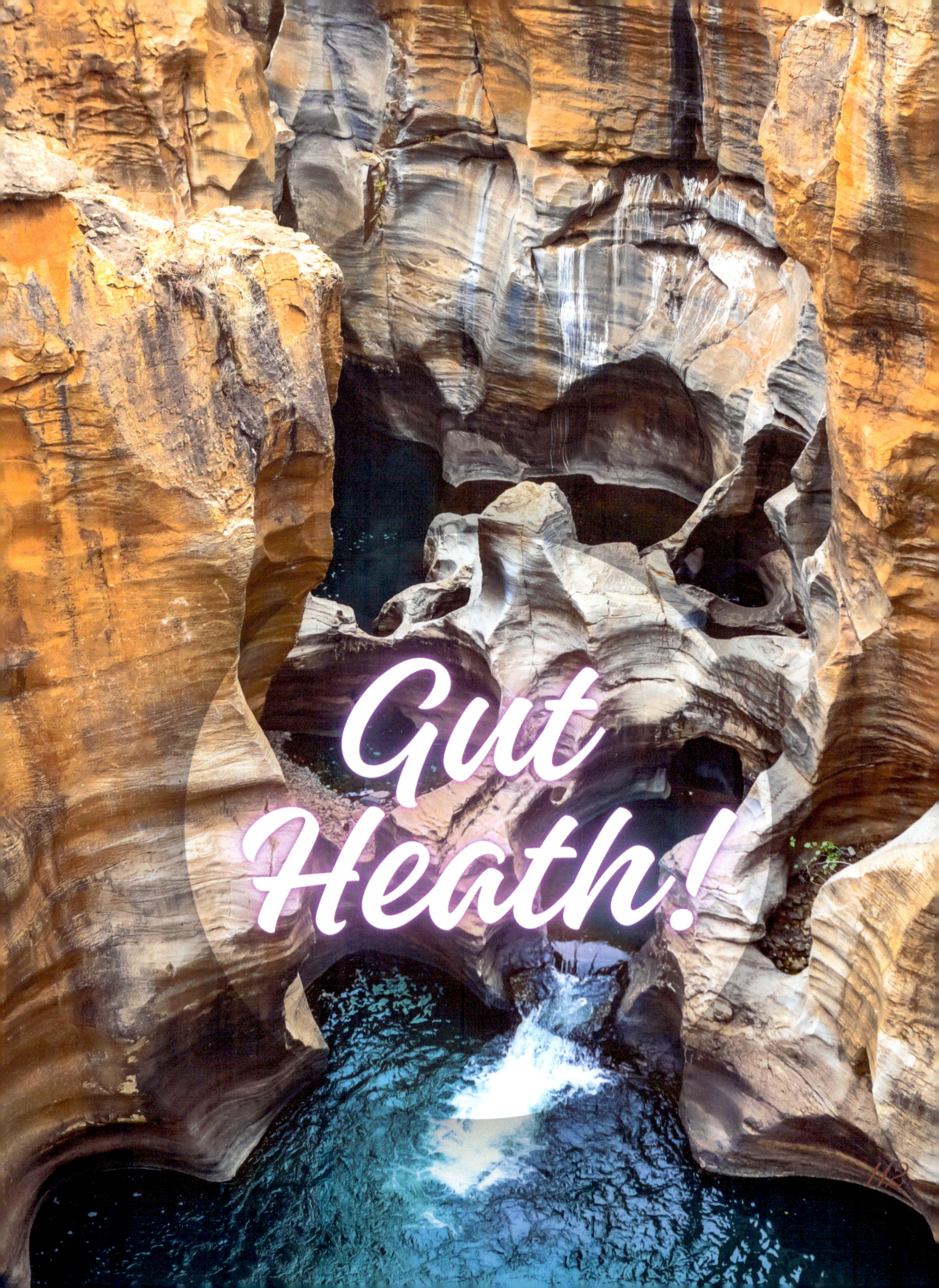

The Power of the Gut Microbiome

Recent nutrition research has shed light on a fascinating and complex ecosystem within us: the gut microbiome. This diverse network of microorganisms, bacteria, fungi, and viruses plays a crucial role in shaping our overall health. While many people associate gut health with digestion, its impact extends far beyond that, influencing immune function, mood, and even weight regulation.

A Hidden World Inside Us

The gut microbiome is estimated to contain around 35,000 different bacterial strains, with the majority residing in the large intestine, particularly the colon. But bacteria aren't limited to just one place; they can also be found in the esophagus, stomach, and small intestine, quietly working behind the scenes to support essential bodily functions.

More Than Just Digestion

The gut isn't just responsible for breaking down food; it's a powerhouse that absorbs nutrients, fuels metabolism, and eliminates waste. As food is processed, the microbiome generates bioactive compounds that can either enhance health or, in some cases, contribute to inflammation. This delicate balance may influence the risk of developing conditions like cardiovascular disease and asthma.

The Link Between Gut and Well-being

Gut health plays a direct role in how we feel, physically and emotionally. When the gut lining is constantly exposed to irritants from diet or environmental factors, its integrity can weaken, leading to chronic low-level inflammation. This type of imbalance is increasingly recognized as a driving force behind a wide range of disorders.

Taking care of our gut means more than just eating well; it's about cultivating an environment where beneficial microbes thrive, promoting better digestion, stronger immunity, and even a more balanced mood. As research continues to explore the microbiome's vast influence, one thing is clear: gut health is key to overall wellness.

EASY SAUERKRAUT:

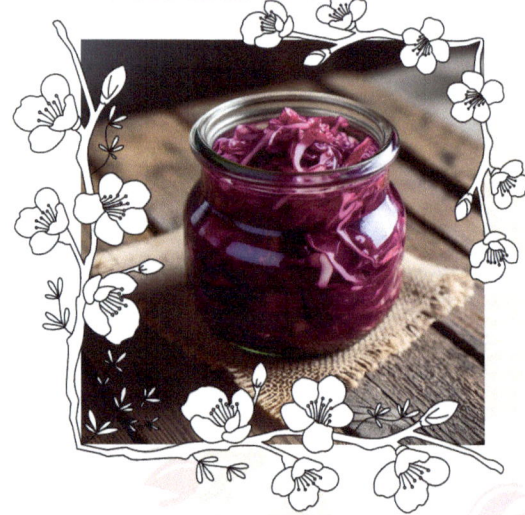

Topping the chart of gut-friendly goodies are those fermented delights, jam-packed with probiotics, the tiny live heroes of health! These microscopic marvels work wonders when they hit your system in the right amount. But wait, there's a twist! To unleash their full superpowers, they need their trusty sidekicks, prebiotics, those sneaky, non-digestible fibers that act as their fuel. Together, they're like a dynamic duo, balancing your gut's ecosystem, boosting digestion, and sprinkling wonders on your well-being. So, dive into tasty treats like yogurt, kefir, sauerkraut, kimchi, and kombucha, and pair them with prebiotic all-stars like garlic, onions, bananas, and asparagus. This culinary combo can turbocharge your digestive health and fortify your immune fortress!

ALL YOU'LL NEED:

- fresh, organic purple cabbage
- High-quality sea salt is ideal, as iodized salt can hinder fermentation.

INSTRUCTIONS:

1. Remove the outer leaves and rinse the cabbage. Cut it into quarters and slice it finely.

2. In a large mixing bowl, take your freshly chopped cabbage and sprinkle 1 to 3 tablespoons of high-quality sea salt over it, adjusting the amount based on your personal preference for saltiness. Using your hands, gently massage the cabbage for about 10 minutes, applying enough pressure to break down the cell walls. This process will help the cabbage become tender while simultaneously releasing its natural juices. For an enjoyable experience, put on your favorite show or podcast to keep you entertained during this hands-on task. You'll know you're done when the cabbage is noticeably softer and has created a fragrant, salty brine at the bottom of the bowl.

3. Transfer the cabbage to your jars, packing it tightly while ensuring it stays submerged in its brine. Place a cabbage leaf on top and push down, leaving some space at the top. Seal the jars and place them in a cool, dark spot (65°F to 75°F) for a day, ensuring the cabbage remains submerged. You can use the bottom of a spoon to help keep it down.

5. Once fermented to your liking (one day works for me), move the jars to the refrigerator. Enjoy your homemade sauerkraut in various dishes for a tasty, nutritious boost!

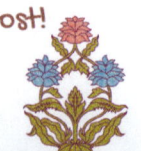

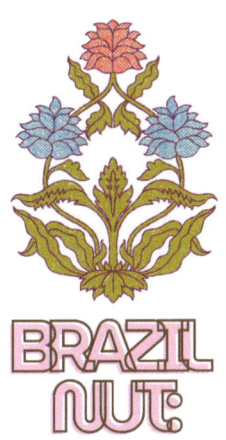

BRAZIL NUT

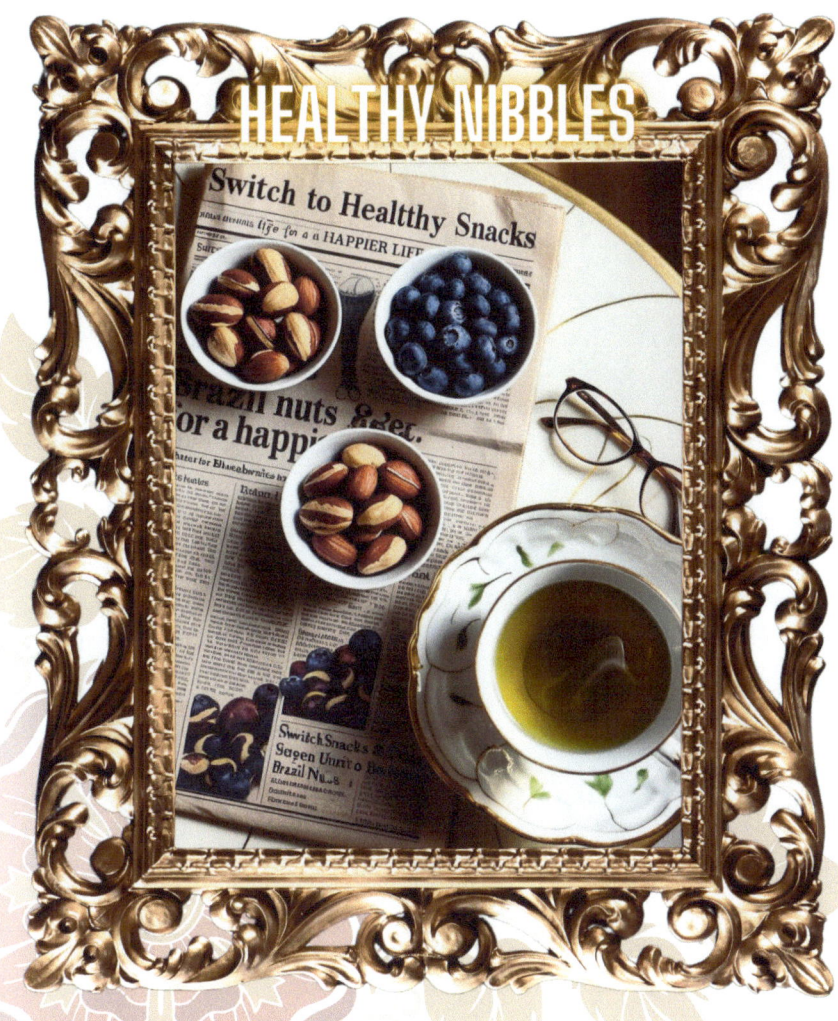

Honestly, growing up, I never heard of Brazil Nut, but illness happened, and we were introduced. I was dealing with thyroid problems, and after doing some research, I found out that Brazil nuts are packed with selenium, which I was lacking. It felt frustrating not having enough of this in my system! It was especially tough because it slowed down my metabolism, and I ended up gaining over 15 pounds.

The recommended amount is three nuts a day, but let me tell you, these little guys have the perfect texture and taste, and stopping at just three is pretty hard!

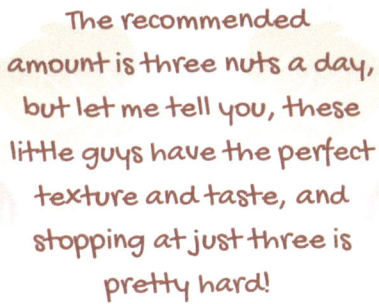

This food item improves focus, promotes a feeling of fullness and heart health, boosts immunity, aids thyroid function, and protects the body from oxidative damage and stress. It is an excellent source of magnesium and phosphorus which are essential for various bodily functions. Magnesium is crucial for energy production, nerve function, and bone health.

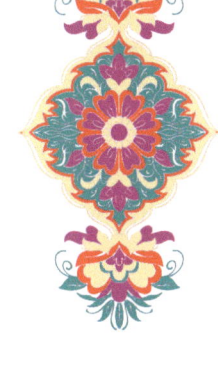

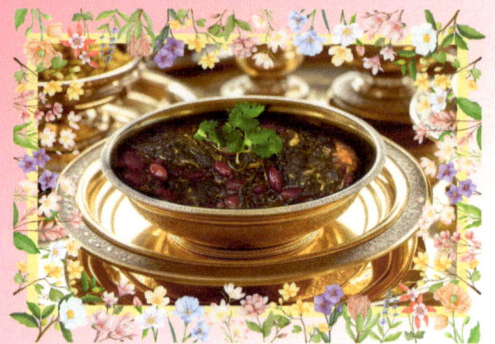

Easy Vegan Sabzi:

Vegan Sabzi is a scrumptious, plant-powered delight that channels the heart of classic sabzi! Bursting with flavors and textures, it's like a cozy hug on a plate.

Ingredients:

- ½ cup avocado oil
- 1 large organic yellow onion, thinly sliced
- 2 tablespoons minced garlic
- 1 tablespoon ground turmeric
- 1 bag (about 10 oz) of pre-washed baby spinach
- 1 bunch of fresh cilantro, rinsed and roughly chopped
- 1 bunch of scallions, washed and finely sliced
- ¼ teaspoon cayenne pepper (adjust to taste)
- 2 tablespoons additional minced garlic
- 2 large ripe tomatoes, diced into small cubes
- ½ cup filtered water
- 3 cups precooked kidney beans, rinsed & drained
- 1 bunch of fresh dill, rinsed and chopped
- 2 tablespoons organic tomato paste
- 2 teaspoons vegan organic bouillon paste

Instructions:

1. Begin by heating a large stainless steel pot over medium heat. Once the pot is hot, add the avocado oil and allow it to warm for about a minute. Next, incorporate the sliced onions, reducing the heat to low. Cover the pot and let the onions sauté gently for 4 to 5 minutes, allowing them to soften.

2. After the onions have softened, uncover the pot, raise the heat to medium-high, and stir the onions frequently until they develop a beautiful caramelized color, which should take around 5-7 minutes.

3. Stir in the minced garlic and sauté for another minute until fragrant. Then, add the ground turmeric along with freshly ground black pepper to taste, mixing well to incorporate the spices.

4. Gradually add the greens to the pot, begin with half of the baby spinach, cilantro, scallions, and dill. Cover the pot, and once the greens begin to wilt, add the remaining greens. Sprinkle in the cayenne pepper, lower the heat to low, and cover partially. Let the mixture simmer gently for about 30 minutes, stirring occasionally.

5. While the greens are cooking, heat a separate medium-sized pan over low heat. Add a splash of avocado oil, then add the diced tomatoes. Cover the pan and let the tomatoes cook for 3 to 5 minutes, allowing them to release their juices. Remove the lid and increase the heat to medium-high, frying the tomatoes uncovered for an additional 3 minutes, stirring occasionally, until they are softened.

6. Stir in the tomato paste and cook on low, stirring frequently until the paste begins to stick to the bottom of the pan (about 5 minutes). This will help deepen the flavors without burning it. Pour in the filtered water, using a spatula to scrape up any bits stuck to the bottom.

Continue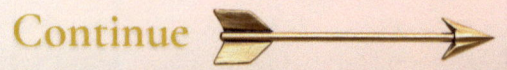

6. Stir in the tomato paste and cook on low, stirring frequently until the paste begins to stick to the bottom of the pan (about 5 minutes). This will help deepen the flavors without burning it. Pour in the filtered water, using a spatula to scrape up any bits stuck to the bottom.

7. Add the vegan bouillon paste, followed by the rinsed kidney beans. Allow the mixture to cook together for about 5 minutes until everything is heated through. Once done, remove from heat and set aside.

8. When the greens in the pot are fully cooked and have reduced significantly in volume, gently fold in the kidney bean mixture, being careful not to mash the beans. Allow everything to cook together for an additional 5 minutes to meld the flavors.

9. Serve your vibrant dish in a deep traditional bowl that celebrates your culinary prowess. Enjoy the delightful combination of flavors and textures, and relish the satisfaction of creating a wholesome and nourishing meal.

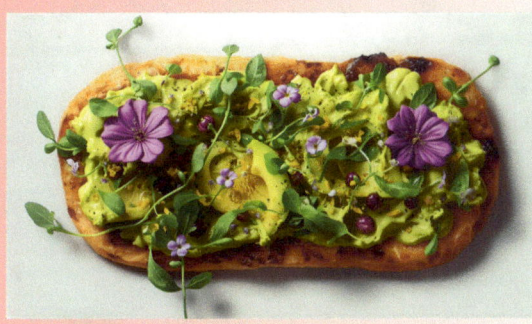

Soft, tangy whole-wheat naan gets a kaleidoscopic makeover—swirled with superfood colors, studded with seeds, and ready in under 30 minutes.

Super Swirl Naan: A Vibrant Wellness Twist

For the Swirl

- 2 tbsp beet juice (or puréed roasted beets)
- 1 tbsp spinach purée
- ½ tsp turmeric powder

Wellness Spark Sprinkles

- 1 tsp black sesame seeds
- 1 tsp chia seeds
- Pinch of crushed red pepper

Ingredients

- 1 cup whole-wheat flour
- ½ cup plain Greek yogurt
- 2 tbsp warm water
- ¼ tsp sea salt
- ½ tsp baking powder
- 1 tsp olive oil (plus extra for cooking)

Instructions:

1. Whisk flour, salt, and baking powder in a bowl.
2. Stir in yogurt and water until a rough dough forms.
3. Knead on a floured surface for 2–3 minutes until smooth and elastic.
4. Divide dough into three equal balls; cover with a damp cloth and rest 5 minutes.
5. Meanwhile, mix each ball with one swirl color:
   - Roll out plain dough; transfer to a plate.
   - Flatten beet dough atop plain, then fold and roll to marbled pink.
   - Repeat with spinach and turmeric dough for green and golden streaks.
6. Heat a nonstick skillet over medium; brush lightly with oil.
7. Cook each swirl-patterned naan 2 minutes per side, pressing gently until puffed and dotted with char.
8. While hot, brush with a little olive oil and sprinkle Spark Sprinkles over the surface.

Fun Serving Ideas: Layer with smashed avocado, lemon zest, and microgreens.

117

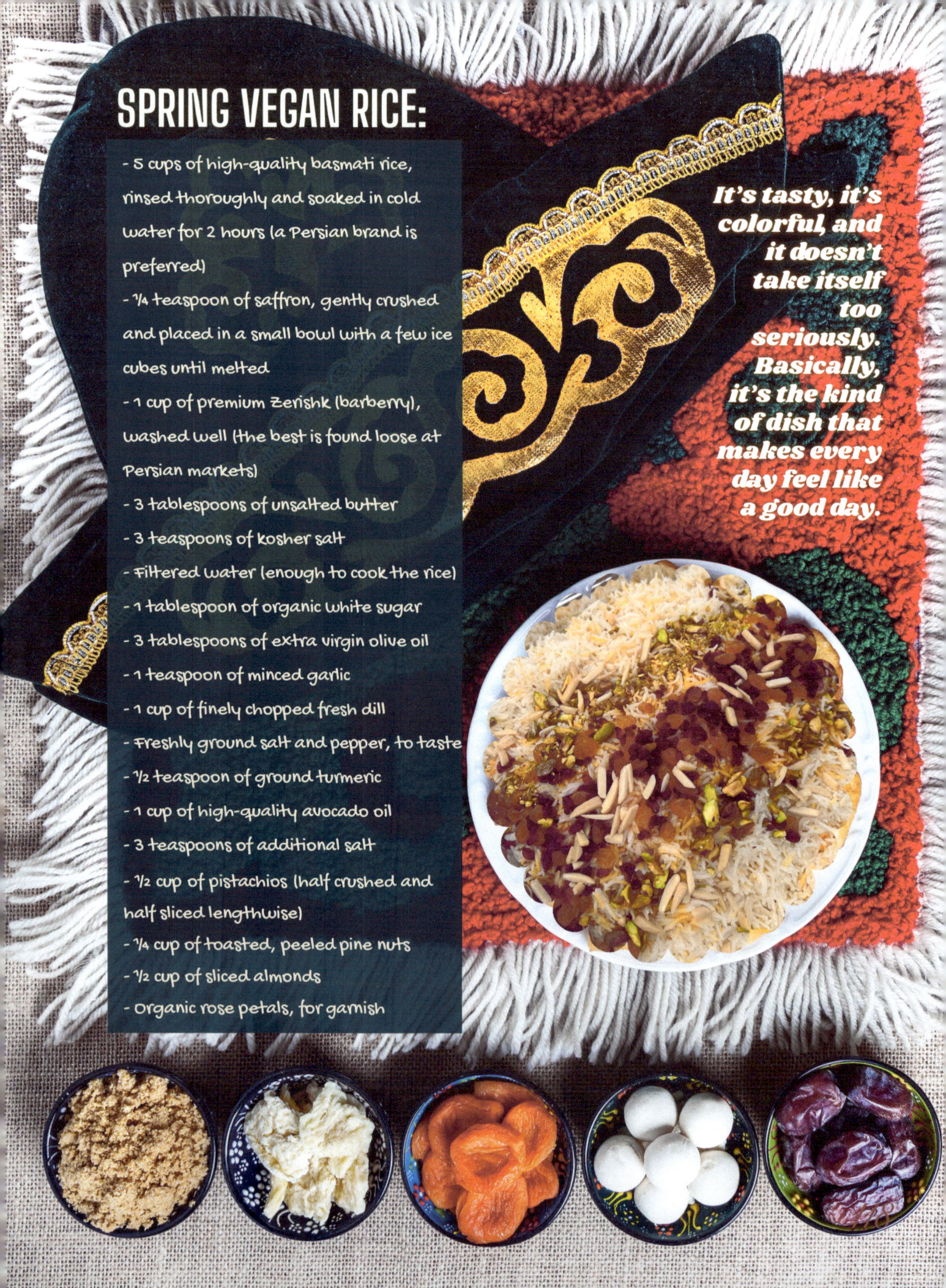

SPRING VEGAN RICE:

- 5 cups of high-quality basmati rice, rinsed thoroughly and soaked in cold water for 2 hours (a Persian brand is preferred)
- ¼ teaspoon of saffron, gently crushed and placed in a small bowl with a few ice cubes until melted
- 1 cup of premium Zereshk (barberry), washed well (the best is found loose at Persian markets)
- 3 tablespoons of unsalted butter
- 3 teaspoons of kosher salt
- Filtered water (enough to cook the rice)
- 1 tablespoon of organic white sugar
- 3 tablespoons of extra virgin olive oil
- 1 teaspoon of minced garlic
- 1 cup of finely chopped fresh dill
- Freshly ground salt and pepper, to taste
- ½ teaspoon of ground turmeric
- 1 cup of high-quality avocado oil
- 3 teaspoons of additional salt
- ½ cup of pistachios (half crushed and half sliced lengthwise)
- ¼ cup of toasted, peeled pine nuts
- ½ cup of sliced almonds
- Organic rose petals, for garnish

It's tasty, it's colorful, and it doesn't take itself too seriously. Basically, it's the kind of dish that makes every day feel like a good day.

INSTRUCTIONS

1. PREPARE THE ZERISHK

Melt butter in a medium pot and add the washed Zerishk. Sauté over medium heat for 3 to 5 minutes until the berries soften and release their aroma. Turn off the heat, sprinkle in sugar, then pour in the saffron water. Cover partially and let the flavors meld gently.

2. SAUTÉ THE DILL

In another pot, heat olive oil until shimmering. Add minced garlic and cook until golden bronze, careful not to burn. Stir in chopped dill, season with salt, pepper, and turmeric. Add ¼ cup water, cover partially, and set aside.

3. COOK THE RICE

Drain the soaked basmati rice and place it in a wide pot. Add 3 teaspoons salt and avocado oil. Pour in filtered water to cover the rice by an inch. Cover and bring to a boil over high heat.

4. STEAM THE RICE

Once boiling, uncover and gently push rice from edges to center to keep it loose. When water mostly evaporates, reduce heat to low. Scoop 6 cups of rice and set aside. Make holes in remaining rice, cover with a clean towel and lid—avoid scorching the towel—and steam (Dumlah) for 10 minutes. Let rest 5 minutes with heat off.

5. COMBINE FLAVORED RICE

Fold half the reserved rice into the Zerishk mixture and the other half into the dill mixture. Cover both pots with towels and steam on very low heat for 10 minutes to allow flavors to infuse.

6. ASSEMBLE THE DISH

Fluff the plain rice gently in a large serving dish. Lay down two-inch lines of Zerishk rice spaced about 4 inches apart, then repeat with the dill rice, creating a beautiful tri-color presentation of white, yellow, and green.

7. GARNISH AND SERVE

Top with crushed pistachios, toasted pine nuts, sliced almonds, and rose petals for a fragrant, elegant finish. Serve immediately and enjoy this Persian-inspired dish.

RELATIONSHIPS:

Since the beginning of time,
survival did not belong to the strongest; it belonged to
the connected. The fires of our ancestors burned brightest when many
gathered around them, when hands reached for hands, when voices
intertwined in stories that refused to be forgotten.

And even now, in this age of endless distractions, our souls know the truth:
we do not merely crave connection, we require it. It is the quiet gravity
pulling two strangers toward understanding, the invisible thread weaving
through generations, the pure electricity in a single look that says, I see you. I
know you. You are not alone.
Because what are we, without each other? Science echoes what hearts have
always whispered; human bonds heal. They lower stress, strengthen our
bodies, sharpen our minds. Love is not just emotion; it is medicine. It is
sanctuary. It is the breath between chaos and calm.

Loneliness, though, loneliness starves us. Studies show that isolation weighs
on the body like sickness, that it can be as lethal as smoking fifteen cigarettes
a day. But the worst part? Loneliness convinces us that connection is out of
reach, that we are somehow separate from the warmth we deserve.
Yet here's the truth: we are meant for each other.

So think of laughter crashing like waves against the quiet. Think of the steady
weight of a hand gripping yours in the darkness. Think of the way a single act
of kindness, a glance, a word, a touch, can change the entire course of a life.
Connection is not just instinct, it is the essence of being human. And in a
world that is drowning in noise but starving for depth, the call to build
something real has never been louder.

Cling to it. Ignite it. Defend it. Because in the end, it is not success,
or wealth, or knowledge that makes us whole... it is each other.

FAMILY: NO FILTER

The very word family opens
a vast chamber within me, echoing with
memory, duty, and love. It is at once a crown
and a weight-glorious to carry, heavy to bear.
Family is the raised voices that rattle the walls, the
slammed doors that sting, and the reconciliations that
soften us again. It is the drama we can't escape,
because it is written into our blood.

And yet, beneath the noise, family is the hearth. It is
the laughter that erupts in the middle of a meal, the
quiet hand that finds yours when the world feels too
sharp, the unspoken promise that no matter how far
you fall, someone will be there to lift you. It is the
late-night phone call answered without hesitation, the
soup made when you're too weak to stand, the
embrace that says, you are safe here, you are still ours.

Family is where we are most unguarded-messy,
imperfect, unpolished-and still loved. It is the storm
and the shelter, the quarrel and the embrace, the ache
and the balm. It is the place that teaches us how to
fight, how to forgive, and how to belong.

In the end, family is everything: the chaos that tests us,
the love that saves us, the circle we return to again and
again. It is the drama that makes us human, and the
warmth that makes us whole

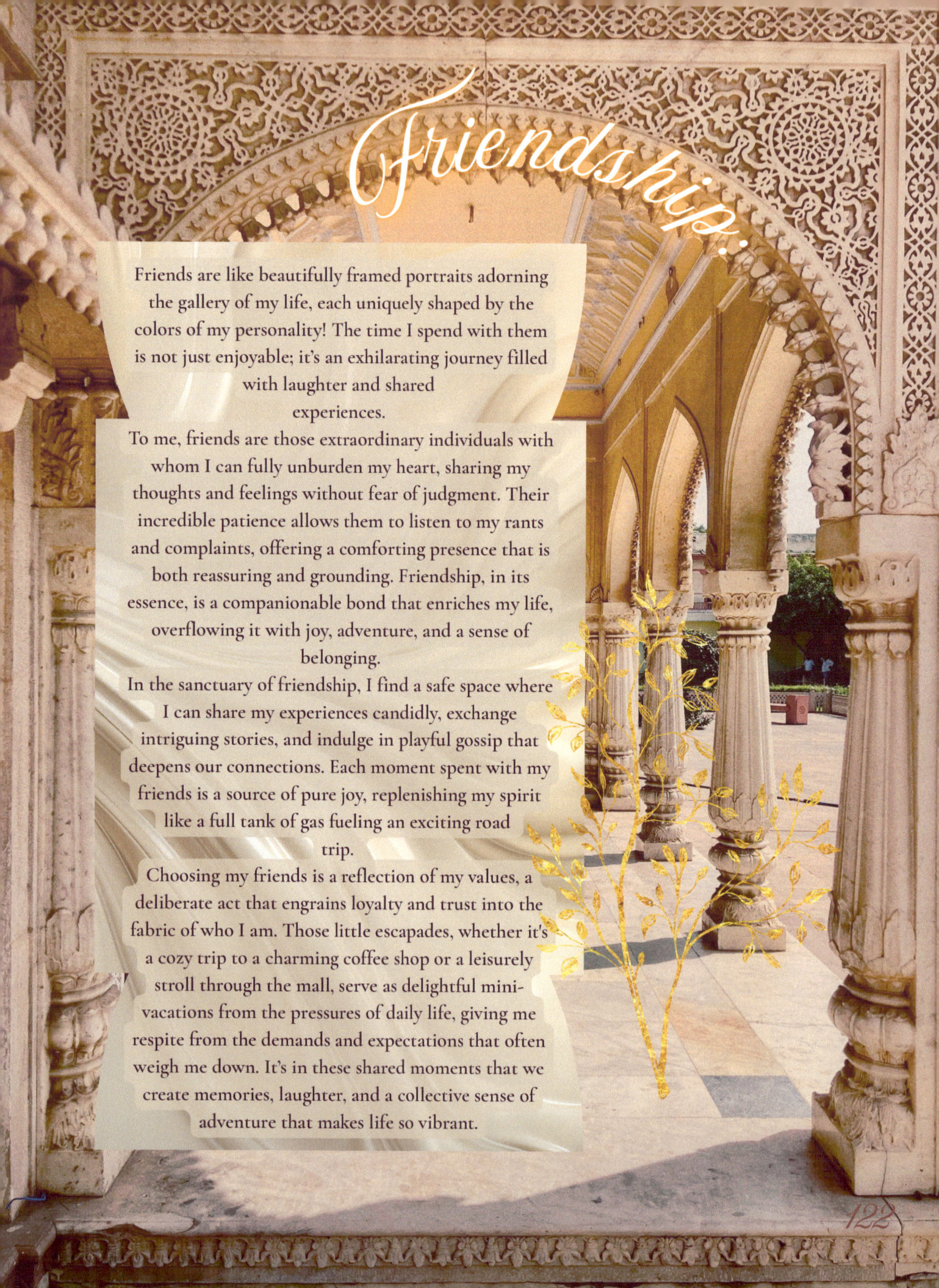

Friendship.

Friends are like beautifully framed portraits adorning the gallery of my life, each uniquely shaped by the colors of my personality! The time I spend with them is not just enjoyable; it's an exhilarating journey filled with laughter and shared experiences.

To me, friends are those extraordinary individuals with whom I can fully unburden my heart, sharing my thoughts and feelings without fear of judgment. Their incredible patience allows them to listen to my rants and complaints, offering a comforting presence that is both reassuring and grounding. Friendship, in its essence, is a companionable bond that enriches my life, overflowing it with joy, adventure, and a sense of belonging.

In the sanctuary of friendship, I find a safe space where I can share my experiences candidly, exchange intriguing stories, and indulge in playful gossip that deepens our connections. Each moment spent with my friends is a source of pure joy, replenishing my spirit like a full tank of gas fueling an exciting road trip.

Choosing my friends is a reflection of my values, a deliberate act that engrains loyalty and trust into the fabric of who I am. Those little escapades, whether it's a cozy trip to a charming coffee shop or a leisurely stroll through the mall, serve as delightful mini-vacations from the pressures of daily life, giving me respite from the demands and expectations that often weigh me down. It's in these shared moments that we create memories, laughter, and a collective sense of adventure that makes life so vibrant.

My dearest,
 I once believed I was complete, untouched by longing, untouched by love. My days had rhythm, my nights had peace. I didn't chase romance, didn't ache for vows. I wore my independence with quiet grace, content in the stillness I'd cultivated for myself.

And yet, you arrived, not with noise, not with promises.
 You came like a breeze through open curtains. No grand entrances, no demands. You simply stepped in where space had always waited, your presence settling gently, like something the soul already recognized.
Love did not rush me. It curled beside my silence.

 Your laughter wove into my days like threads I never knew were missing. Your touch didn't hurry, it lingered, respectful, tender. With you, solitude didn't disappear. It softened. It opened. It began to share the room.
I never thought I needed marriage. But love, once revealed, asked for a place to rest.

Marriage became the quiet truth beneath the ordinary, a pot on the stove, your fingers brushing mine as I sliced peaches, the knowing in your eyes when the tea was steeped just enough. It wasn't ceremony. It was steady flame.

And then, quietly, you were gone.
Now the silence is louder.
 I still reach for your hand in the dark. I still turn toward your voice, expecting to find it suspended in the air. But you are not there, and I am left with the ache of discovery that love had reshaped me without my asking.
I was whole before you.
 And yet, without you, I feel tenderly unfinished.
Return to me, love. Not with thunder. Just as you came, gently.

 As if you'd always been here.
 Yours, in every breath, every quiet moment, every hope.

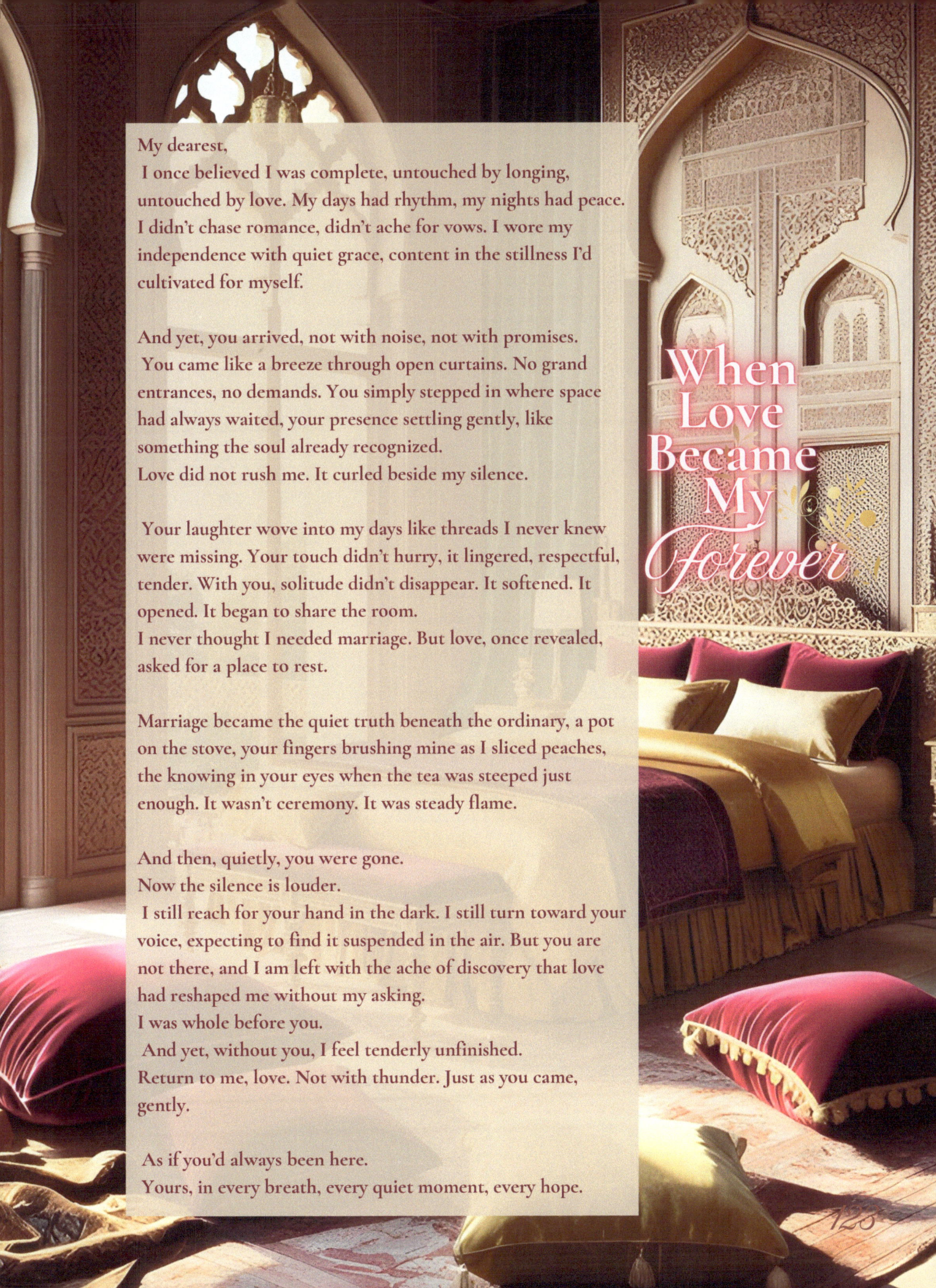

When
Love
Became
My
Forever

Chapli Kabab
Sizzling in Silence

Some memories don't fade.

They rise with the scent of cumin, sizzle beneath the press of my palm. These kababs, spiced and seared, were the ones I made the day your silence felt heavier than usual. I didn't cry. I cooked. I let longing become flavor. With each crusted edge, I remembered you, the way you hovered beside me in the kitchen, the way your laughter made room for mine.

I don't believe food heals everything. But it holds. It carries.

It becomes the thing we return to when words no longer come, when the heart folds inward and the hands take over. This dish, simple, grounding, vibrant, is the one that reminded me I could still nourish myself, even without you.

Chapli kababs, they're called.

Aromatic and bold, named after the Pashto word for "flat," because the flatter they are, the yummier they get. On busy days, I reach for them, letting my outdoor griddle do the work, efficient, generous, sizzling under the open sky.

They pair beautifully with fragrant white rice and silky white sauce.

That combination-warm, tangy, creamy-is more than balanced. It's belonging.

And the next day, the leftovers say something new: sandwiches tucked into pita, layered with creamy hummus and tangy pickles. Comfort, reshaped. Love, repurposed.

This dish is more than a recipe.

It's a memory you can taste.

A devotion that never needed declarations.

A quiet love that still sizzles on the skillet.

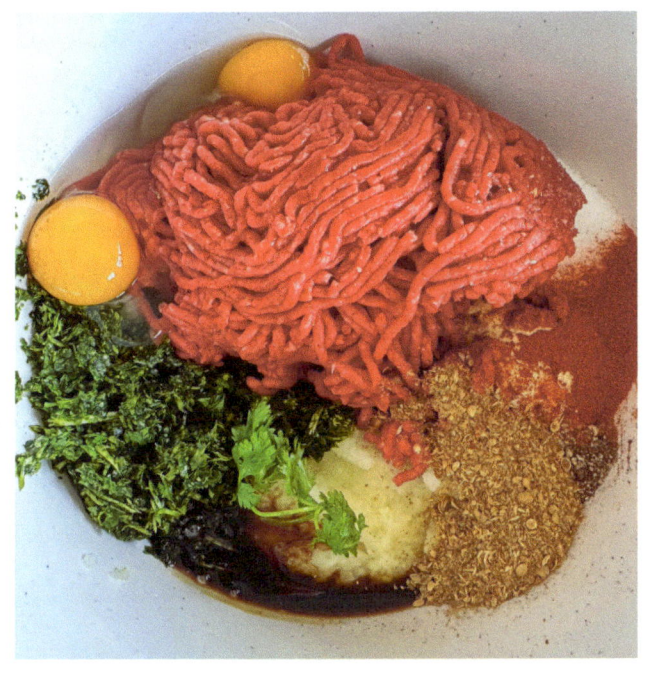
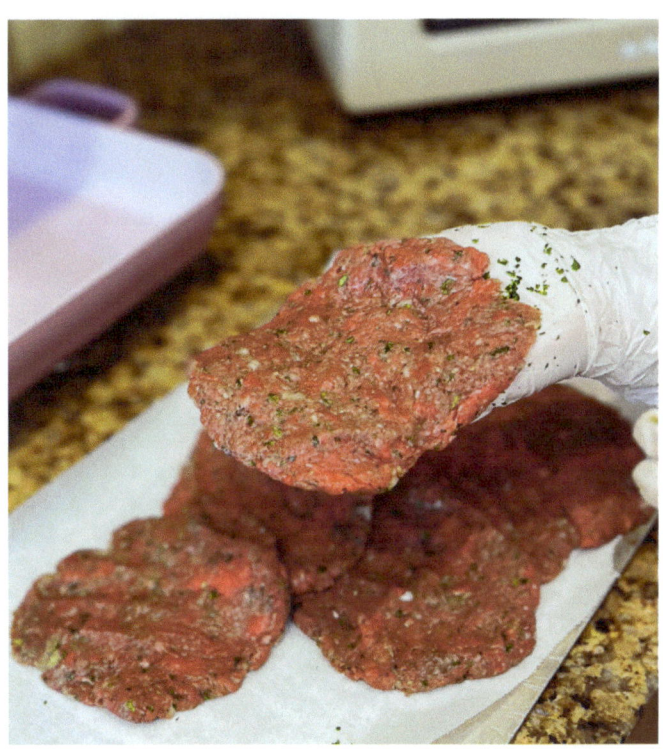
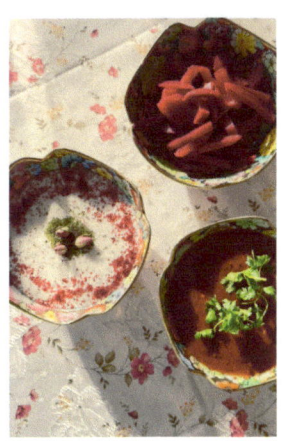
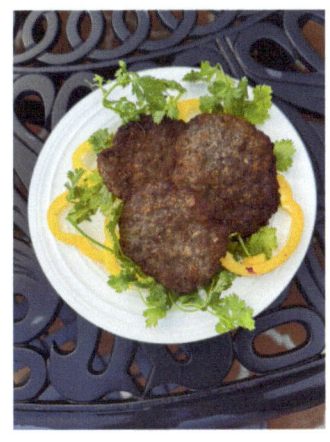
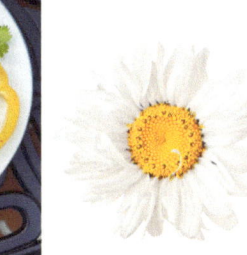
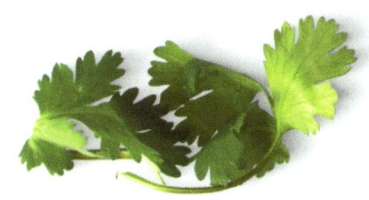
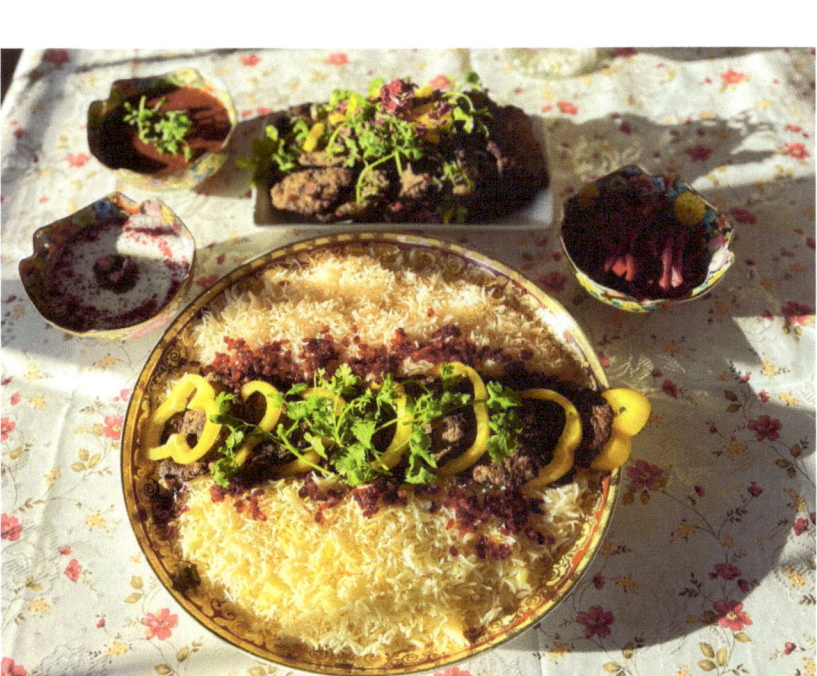
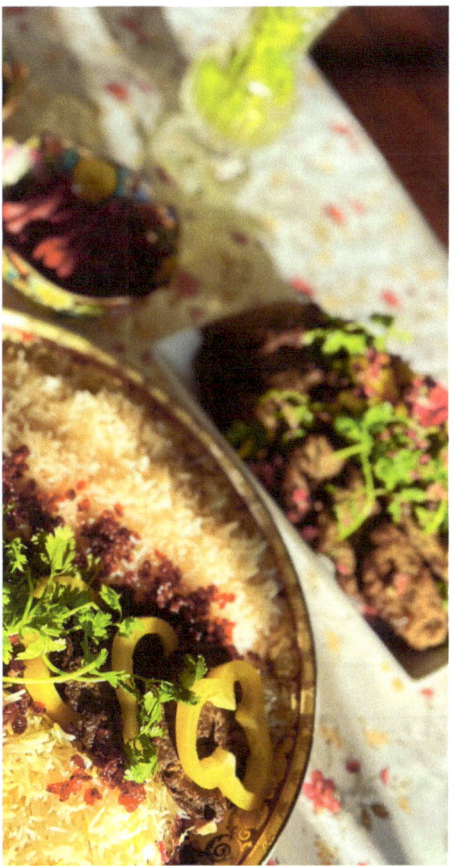

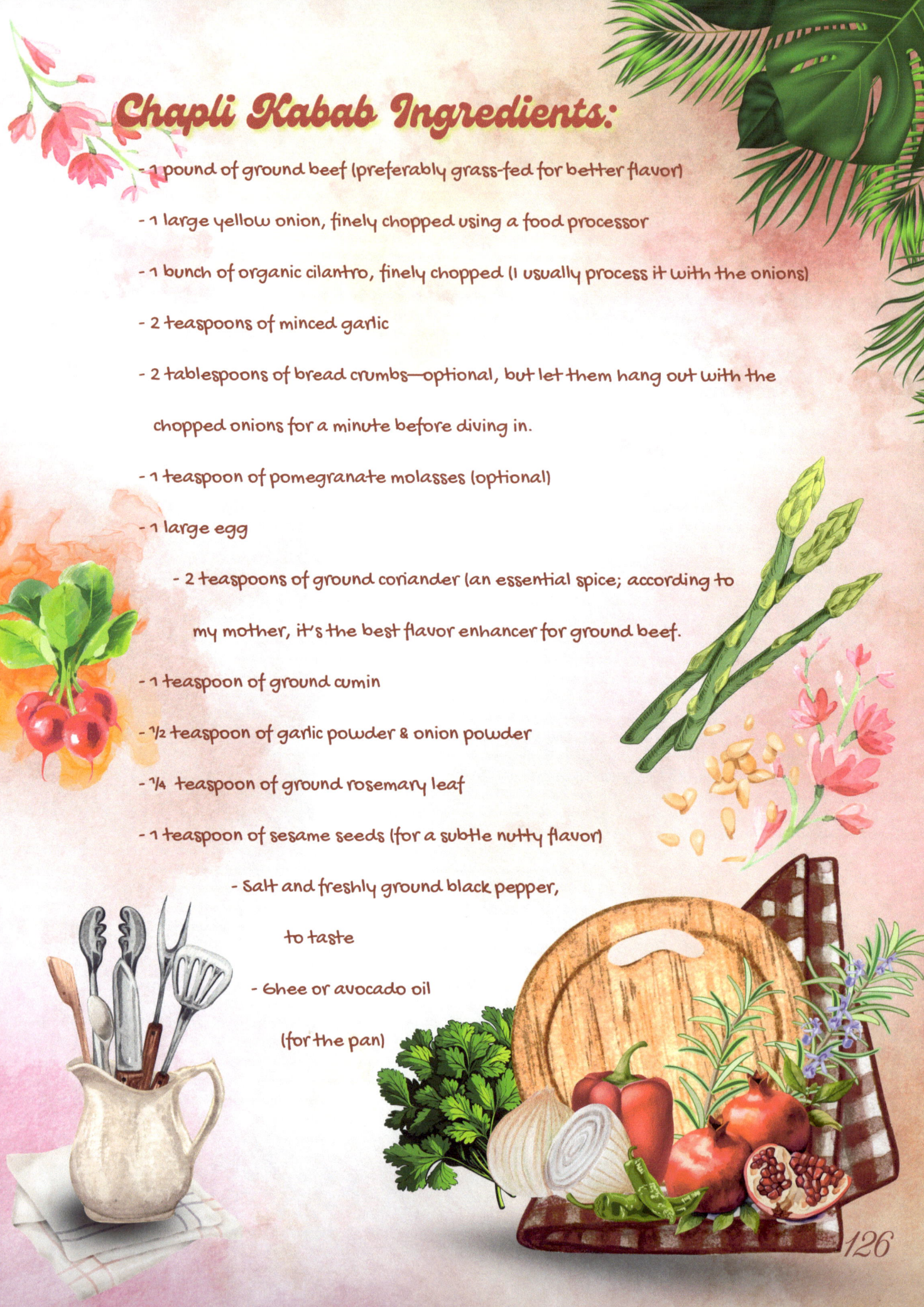

Chapli Kabab Ingredients:

- 1 pound of ground beef (preferably grass-fed for better flavor)

- 1 large yellow onion, finely chopped using a food processor

- 1 bunch of organic cilantro, finely chopped (I usually process it with the onions)

- 2 teaspoons of minced garlic

- 2 tablespoons of bread crumbs—optional, but let them hang out with the

  chopped onions for a minute before diving in.

- 1 teaspoon of pomegranate molasses (optional)

- 1 large egg

- 2 teaspoons of ground coriander (an essential spice; according to

  my mother, it's the best flavor enhancer for ground beef.

- 1 teaspoon of ground cumin

- ½ teaspoon of garlic powder & onion powder

- ¼ teaspoon of ground rosemary leaf

- 1 teaspoon of sesame seeds (for a subtle nutty flavor)

- Salt and freshly ground black pepper,

  to taste

- Ghee or avocado oil

  (for the pan)

INSTRUCTIONS

The spice drapes the air, familiar, like a voice you knew before language.

1. In a large bowl, gather your ingredients: ground meat, crushed coriander, vibrant chili, minced onions, pomegranate molasses. Add everything but the oil.

2. Slide on disposable gloves. Use your hands. Not just to mix, but to remember. Fold, press, blend until the mixture holds, not too tight, not too loose. It should feel like something becoming itself.

3. If time allows, cover with plastic wrap. Let the flavors rest for an hour or two in the fridge. Let them talk. Let them wait.

4. Shape into thin patties, rough around the edges. Don't smooth them out; they weren't meant to be perfect.

5. Preheat a griddle over medium heat, or place a sturdy skillet over medium-high. Add ghee or avocado oil, enough to coat, not drown. When the oil shimmers, it's ready.

6. Sear the patties gently. Five minutes per side, give or take. Listen to the sizzle, it's telling a story. A dark, crisp crust is your cue. Add oil as needed. Don't rush.

7. Once cooked, transfer the patties to a serving platter. Garnish with chopped dill and scallions, and serve alongside grilled tomatoes.

The last patty settles into the platter, edges darkened, imperfect, true.
Oil cools in the pan, no longer urgent.
Steam rises, not just from heat, but from history.
A lesson held in the hands:
some flavors only come through when you
stop trying to fix them.
No words. Just the weight of something returned.
The spice drapes the air; familiar, like a voice
you trusted before it ever spoke.

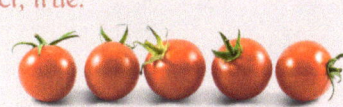
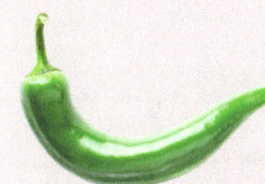

a Heartfelt Note on Love

Every person has their own special "joy button" (okay, most folks do), a hidden switch that lights up their world with happiness, satisfaction, and all those warm fuzzies! This button is wired to unleash a flood of feel-good chemicals like oxytocin, dopamine, and serotonin, boosting bliss and deepening bonds.

Cracking the code on what makes your partner feel truly adored is the secret sauce for a rock-solid relationship. It's all about tuning in, chatting openly, and making a heartfelt effort to vibe with their likes, dreams, and emotional hot spots.

By honing in on this powerful part of your partner's essence, you create a cozy haven where they feel treasured and seen. This mutual understanding not only tightens your connection but also builds a love fortress that can withstand any storm.

Once you master the art of what tickles your partner's fancy, you spark a powerful, intimate connection that paves the way for eternal devotion. When both partners dive into this emotional treasure hunt, they lay the groundwork for a love story bursting with affection, respect, and an unshakeable sense of togetherness. With this newfound wisdom, your partner will feel utterly cherished, and in return, they're forever yours!

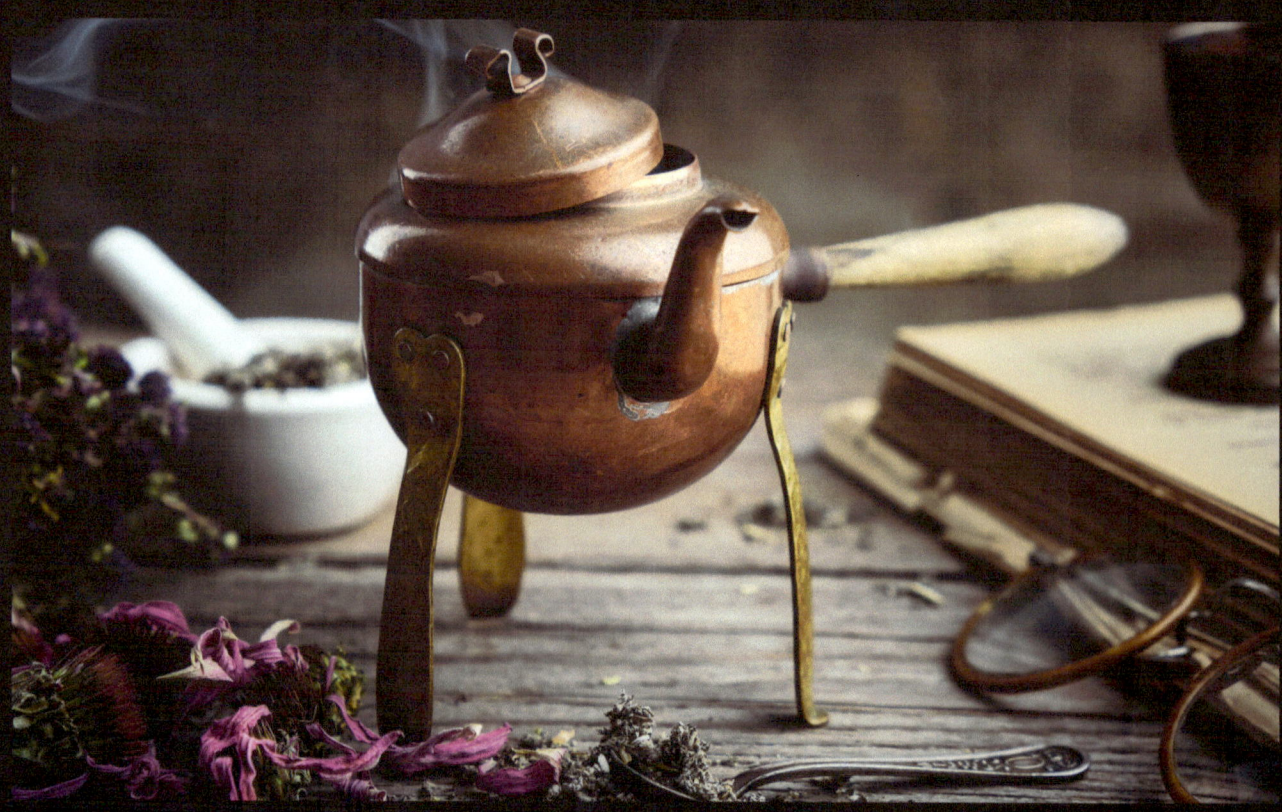

Sweet Trap: Watch What You Buy!

Grocery shopping? Think of it as a red carpet event for your health. Every label is a script, and sugar loves a disguise-fructose, dextrose, corn syrup, maltodextrin. If you're not reading like a detective, you're giving sugar the spotlight it doesn't deserve.

"Sugar-free" and "low-calorie" might sound like wellness royalty, but they often come dressed in artificial sweeteners that blur your instincts and stir up cravings. Less isn't always better-sometimes it's just dressed to deceive. Sweetness should serve you, not seduce you.

Glamour is clarity. Power is choice. When your cart reflects intention, not impulse, you're not just eating; you're editing your legacy.

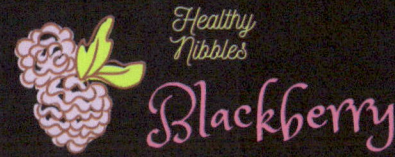

Healthy Nibbles
Blackberry

I'm a card-carrying member of the "Love Your Liver" club, and if you're as fond of your liver as I am, you'll go bananas, or rather, blackberries! These little gems are packed with anthocyanins, those liver-loving superheroes that fend off damage and keep things running smoothly. Plus, they're brain boosters, helping with memory hiccups and giving your heart a fighting chance against cardiovascular villains. With a treasure trove of vitamins C and K, they're like a spa day for your skin, promoting collagen and shielding against sun burns. And let's not forget, they're loaded with manganese, the unsung hero of bone building and wound patching. So, nibble on a handful and bask in that radiant glow!

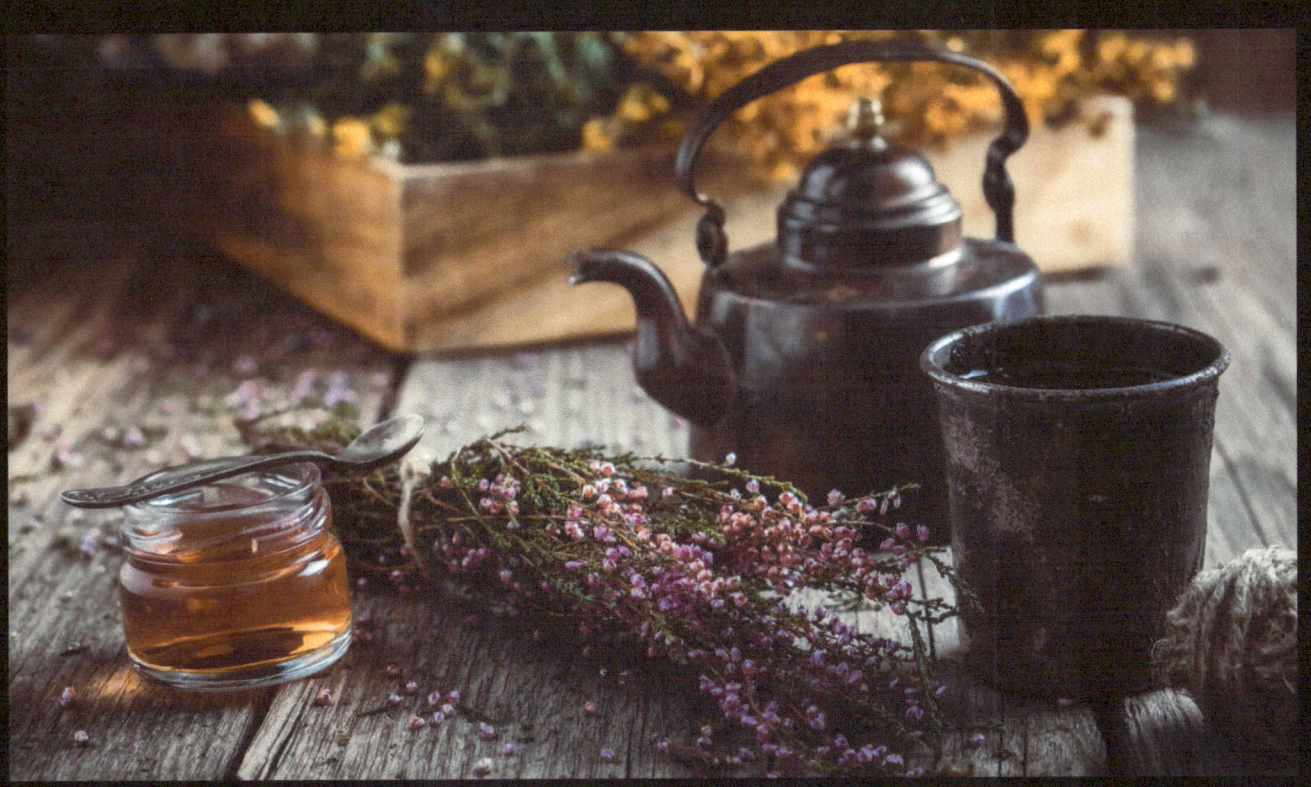

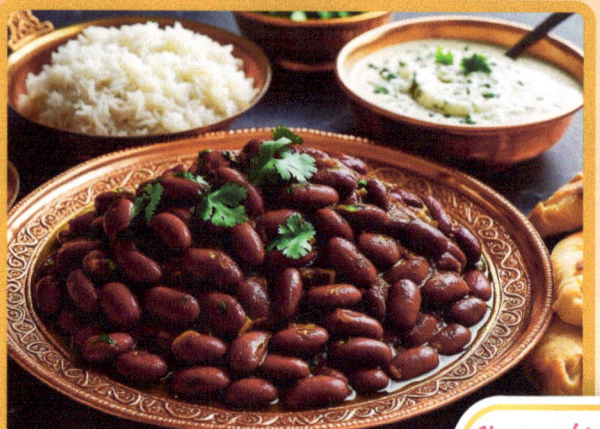

Kidney Bean Qorma

This side dish will elevate the Chapli Kabab and White rice experience to the party level!

- ½ cup of high-quality extra virgin olive oil
- 1 small onion, thinly sliced
- 1 teaspoon minced garlic (about 2-3 cloves)
- 2 ripe tomatoes, chopped (preferably organic)
- 1 teaspoon organic tomato paste
- 1 teaspoon organic vegetable bouillon
- 4 cups of organic cooked kidney beans
- ½ cup of filtered water
- ½ teaspoon ground cumin

1. Begin by heating a stainless steel saucepan over medium heat for about one minute. Once hot, add the olive oil, allowing it to coat the bottom of the pan.

2. Add the thinly sliced onion to the pan. Sauté the onion gently, stirring occasionally, until it becomes soft, translucent, and lightly caramelized, this should take about 5-7 minutes.

3. Once the onions are caramelized, add the minced garlic. Stir and cook for an additional minute until fragrant, being careful not to let the garlic burn.

4. Next, add the chopped tomatoes to the mixture. Stir well to combine, then cover the pan with a lid. Allow the tomatoes to cook on medium-low heat for about 5 minutes until they soften and release their juices.

5. Remove the lid and increase the heat slightly. Continue to cook the tomato mixture, stirring occasionally, until it thickens and the flavors meld, this should take around 5 minutes.

6. Once the tomato mixture reaches your desired consistency, stir in the organic tomato paste and cook for another minute to incorporate the flavors.

7. Add the cooked kidney beans, filtered water, vegetable bouillon, and cumin to the pan, mixing everything thoroughly.

8. Reduce the heat to low and allow the mixture to simmer, partially covered, for about 10 min. Stir occasionally, ensuring the beans are heated through and absorbing the delicious flavors.

9. Serve warm, enjoying the rich flavors of this comforting dish.

Green Sauce Recipe:

Ingredients:

- 1 bunch of organic cilantro, thoroughly washed
- A handful of fresh mint leaves, carefully washed and stems removed
- 1 teaspoon of minced garlic
- 2 cups of creamy organic whole milk plain yogurt for a rich base
- ½ cup of tangy sour cream
- ¼ teaspoon of cayenne pepper for a subtle kick (adjust to taste)
- A pinch of salt to elevate the flavors
- 2 tablespoons of high-quality white vinegar

Instructions:

1. In a blender, combine the cilantro, mint, minced garlic, whole milk yogurt, sour cream, cayenne pepper, salt, and white vinegar.

2. Blend the mixture on high speed until it reaches a smooth, vibrant green consistency. Make sure there are no chunks remaining; the goal is a silky sauce.

3. Taste the sauce and adjust the seasoning if necessary, adding more salt or cayenne pepper according to your preference.

4. Once blended to perfection, transfer the green sauce to a serving bowl or jar.

This green sauce is perfect as a dip for vegetables, a dressing for salads, or a flavorful topping for grilled meats. Enjoy!

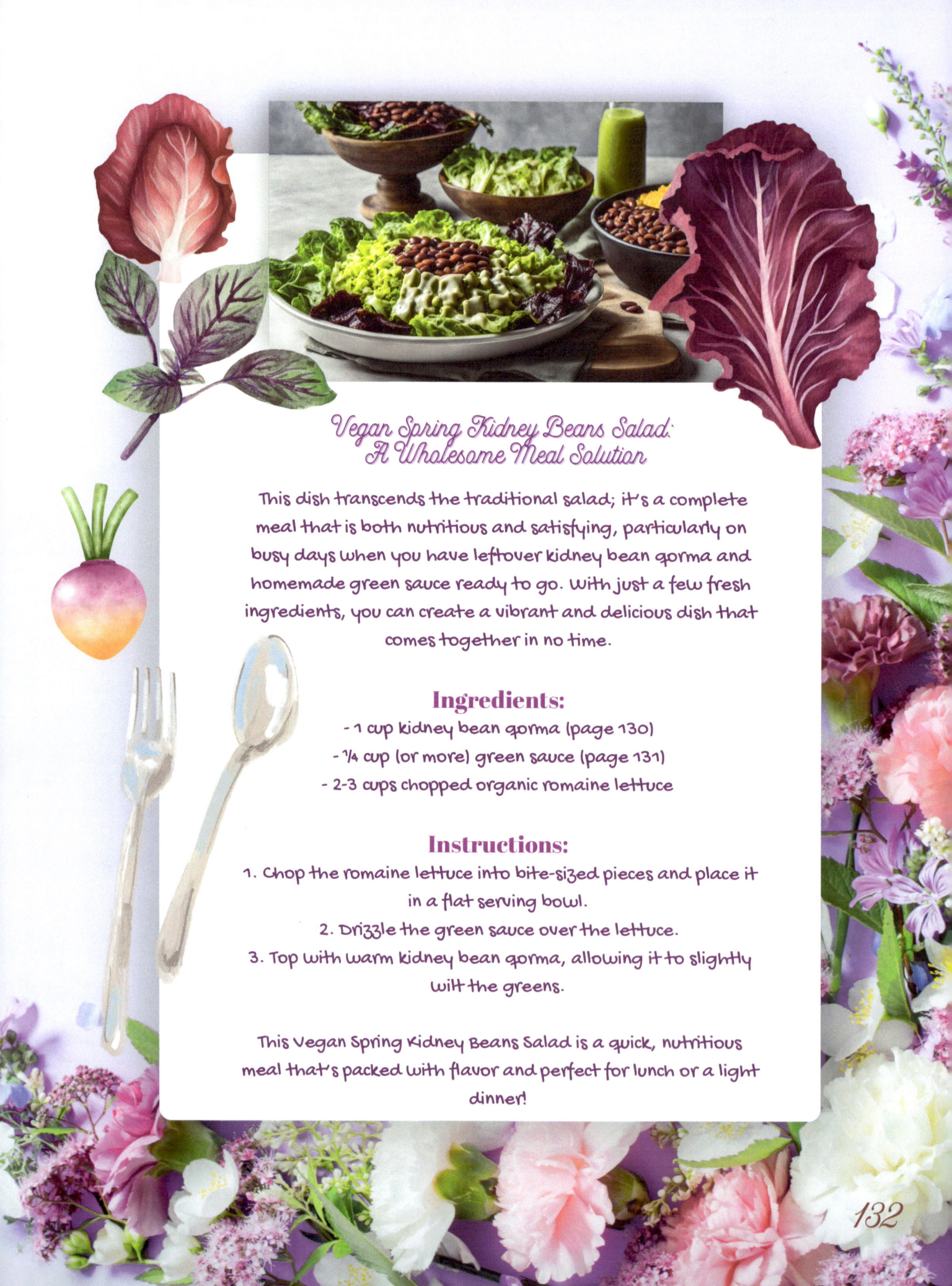

Vegan Spring Kidney Beans Salad: A Wholesome Meal Solution

This dish transcends the traditional salad; it's a complete meal that is both nutritious and satisfying, particularly on busy days when you have leftover kidney bean qorma and homemade green sauce ready to go. With just a few fresh ingredients, you can create a vibrant and delicious dish that comes together in no time.

Ingredients:
- 1 cup kidney bean qorma (page 130)
- ¼ cup (or more) green sauce (page 131)
- 2-3 cups chopped organic romaine lettuce

Instructions:
1. Chop the romaine lettuce into bite-sized pieces and place it in a flat serving bowl.
2. Drizzle the green sauce over the lettuce.
3. Top with warm kidney bean qorma, allowing it to slightly wilt the greens.

This Vegan Spring Kidney Beans Salad is a quick, nutritious meal that's packed with flavor and perfect for lunch or a light dinner!

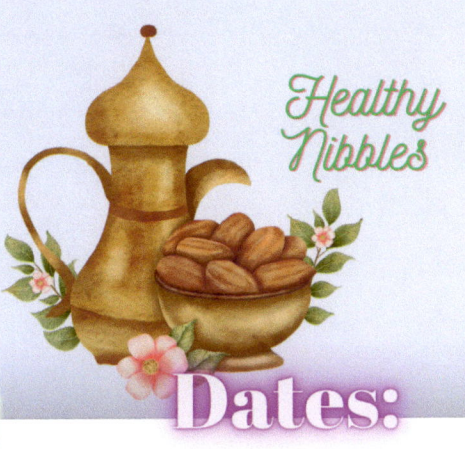

Dates:

Where I grew up, dates were a national sweet treat, so I had the luxury of having so many varieties of dates!

Dates are a great source of various nutrients that support cardiovascular health and improve circulation. I love starting my day with an odd number of these potassium-packed goodies, perfect for your ticker and a sweet swap for those sneaky sugars. Plus, they're fiber-rich, giving your gut a happy dance!

Goji Berries:

Enter the goji berries, the tiny titans of health! These vibrant morsels are immunity-boosting, eye-loving, digestion-friendly powerhouses. Loaded with vitamin A and C, they keep your defenses strong and your vision sharp enough to spot a needle in a haystack. With fiber to keep things moving and iron to turbocharge your blood, goji berries are the real deal!

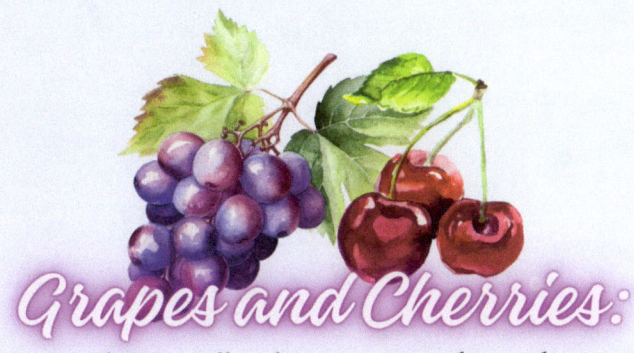

Grapes and Cherries:

Two things I'll always remember about my grandmother (whom we lovingly called Bebe) are her quiet wisdom and her deep love for nature's gifts. She believed in the healing power of simple things: boiling cherry stems into tea to ease kidney stones, and savoring grapes with the kind of joy that made you believe they were truly special.

Bebe was radiant-graceful, sharp-minded, and stunning in every sense. Her intellect stayed luminous until her final breath, and her presence still echoes in the gentle knowledge she passed down.

Grapes, her favorite, are more than sweet indulgence. They're rich in polyphenols that nourish the brain, sharpen cognition, and guard against age-related decline. Their antioxidants and vitamin C help fortify the immune system, while also supporting heart health by easing inflammation and balancing blood pressure.

Cherries, too, carry their own quiet power. Packed with vitamin C and anthocyanins, they help the body fight oxidative stress and inflammation. Their fiber supports digestion and gut health, while their vibrant color hints at the vitality they offer.

In Bebe's world, food was never just sustenance; it was care, knowledge, and love. And in mine, her legacy lives on in every grape I eat and every cherry I steep.

PHYSICAL ACTIVITY:

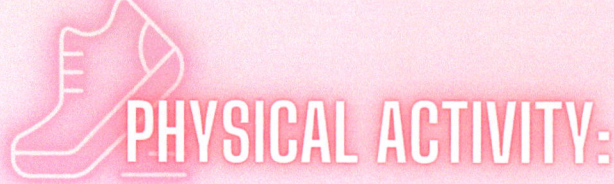

In my 20s, the gym was my escape. No pressure, no hustle culture, just me, building quiet strength and reclaiming self-worth one stretch at a time.

Fast-forward past 40, stress, aging, and an unexpected mirror moment. My skin sagged. My energy felt borrowed. I asked myself, "Wait… where did I go?"

I MADE A SHIFT.

New foods. Mindfulness. And back to the gym, not the cozy home kind, but the real deal. noise echoing off the walls, strangers chasing goals, mirrors reflecting more than just muscle. I didn't return to my old self, I met someone new.

The result? Sleep. Real, delicious, healing sleep. And a body that whispered, thank you.

Then spring showed up like a flirt, warm breezes, blooming sidewalks, scents that made the world feel textured again. I found myself walking farther, running harder, laughing louder. These tiny outdoor habits became mini love letters to myself.

No, I'm not who I was.
I'm something better: evolving, intuitive, radiant in a way I wasn't even chasing.

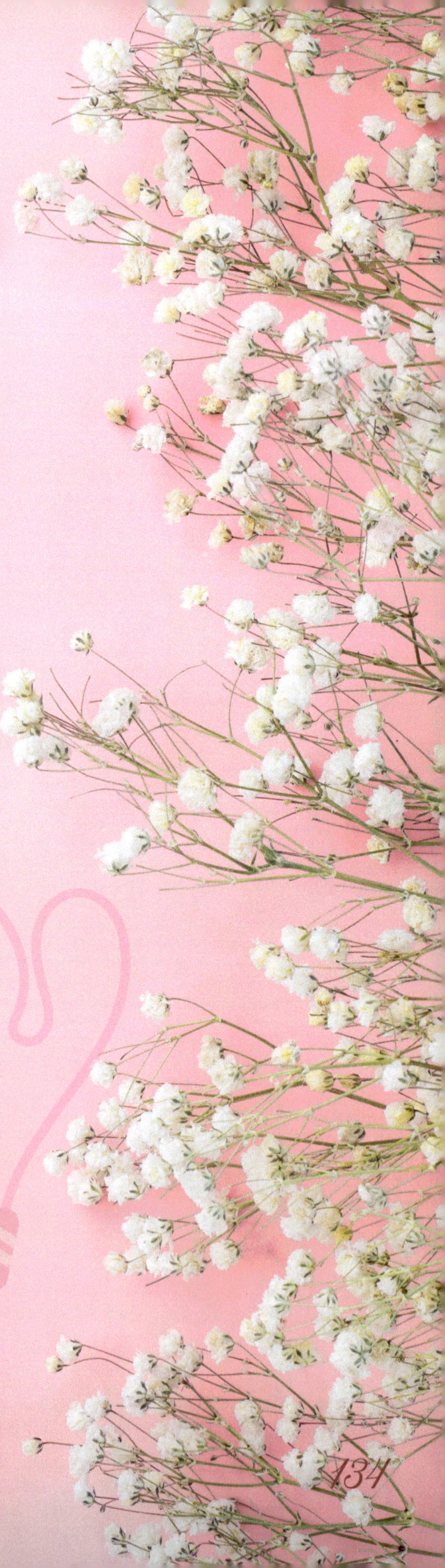

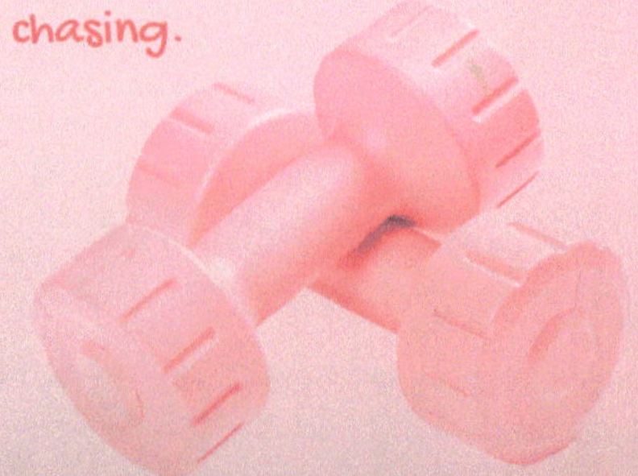

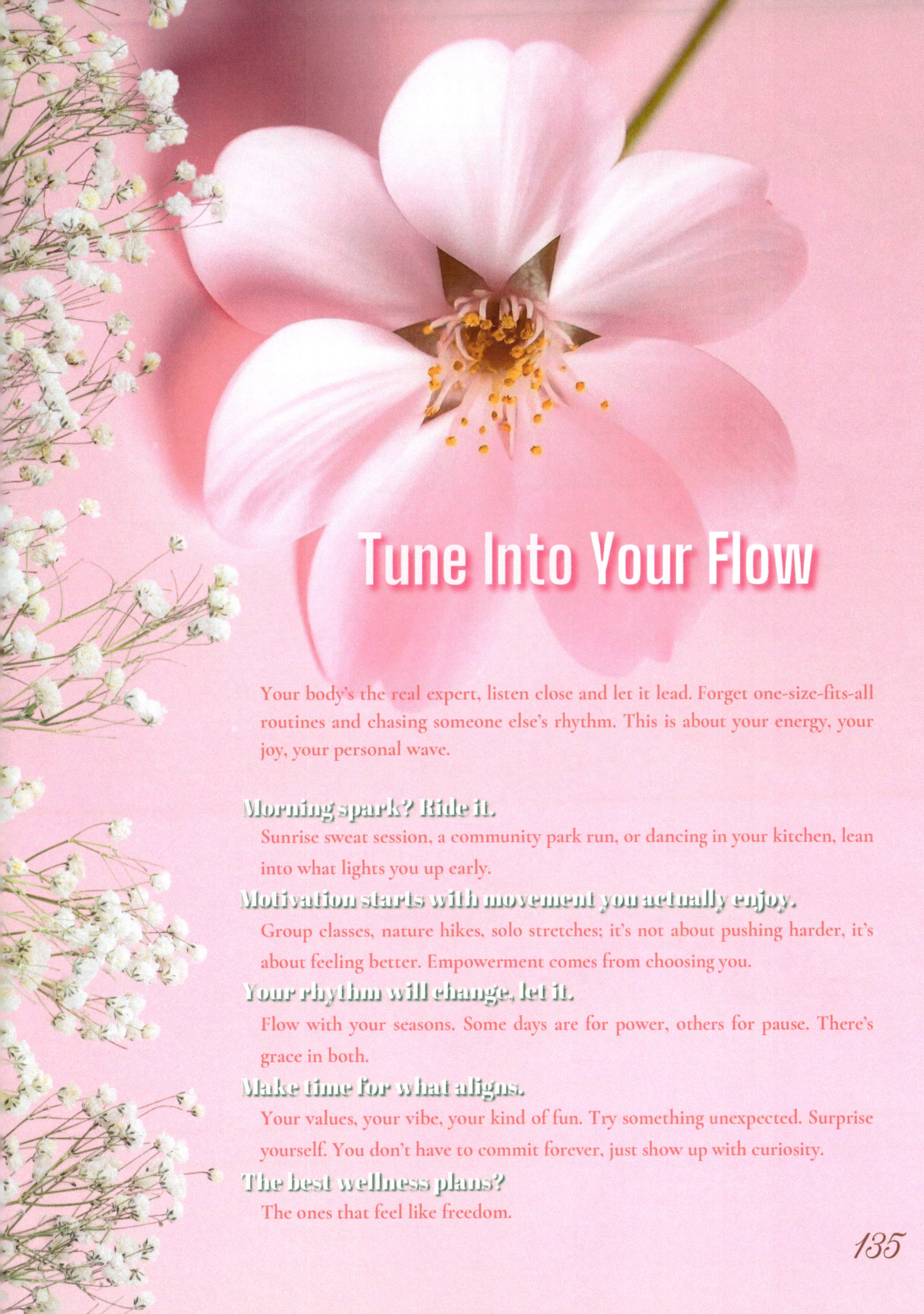

Tune Into Your Flow

Your body's the real expert, listen close and let it lead. Forget one-size-fits-all routines and chasing someone else's rhythm. This is about your energy, your joy, your personal wave.

Morning spark? Ride it.
Sunrise sweat session, a community park run, or dancing in your kitchen, lean into what lights you up early.

Motivation starts with movement you actually enjoy.
Group classes, nature hikes, solo stretches; it's not about pushing harder, it's about feeling better. Empowerment comes from choosing you.

Your rhythm will change, let it.
Flow with your seasons. Some days are for power, others for pause. There's grace in both.

Make time for what aligns.
Your values, your vibe, your kind of fun. Try something unexpected. Surprise yourself. You don't have to commit forever, just show up with curiosity.

The best wellness plans?
The ones that feel like freedom.

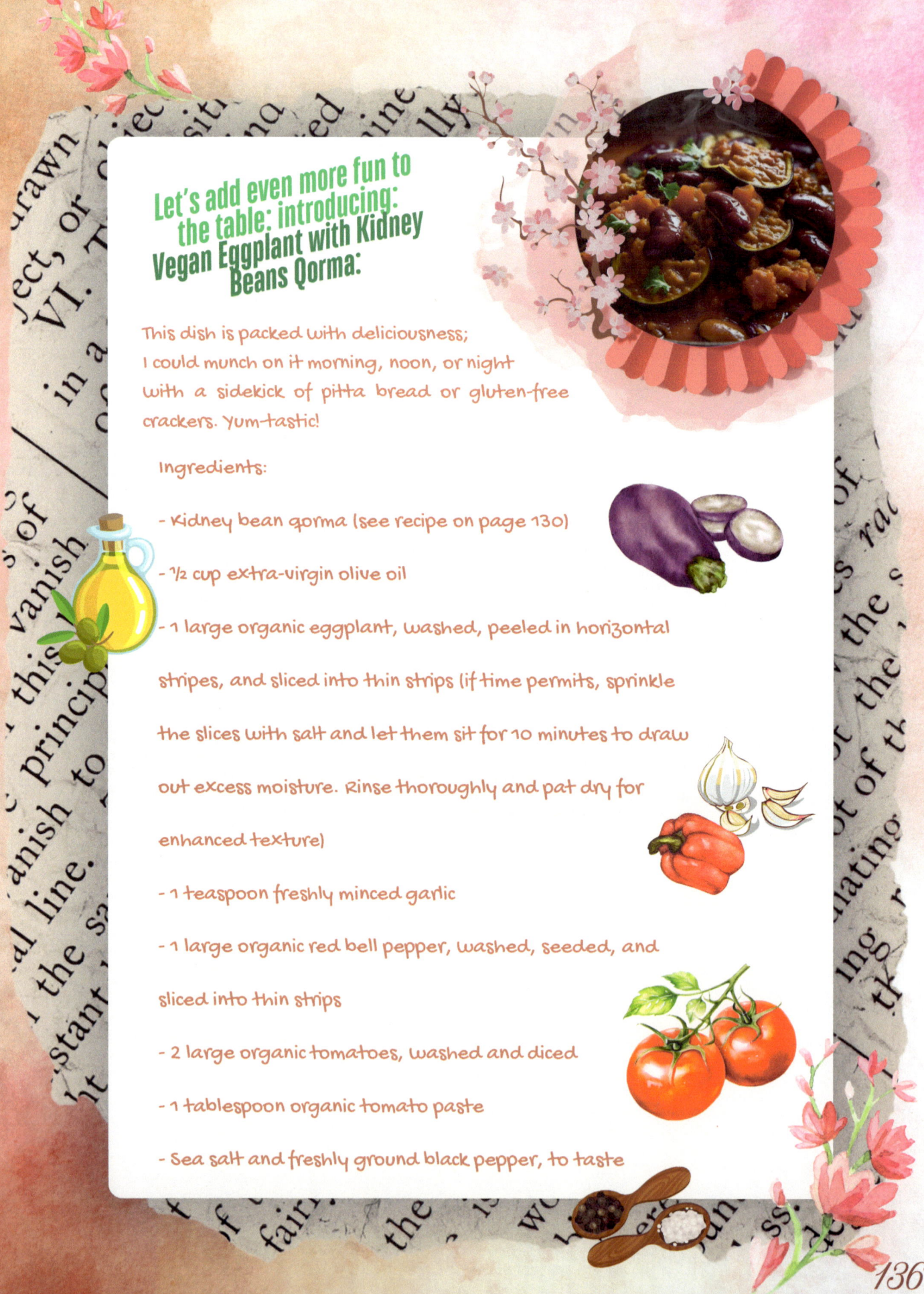

Let's add even more fun to the table: introducing: Vegan Eggplant with Kidney Beans Qorma:

This dish is packed with deliciousness; I could munch on it morning, noon, or night with a sidekick of pitta bread or gluten-free crackers. Yum-tastic!

Ingredients:

- Kidney bean qorma (see recipe on page 130)

- ½ cup extra-virgin olive oil

- 1 large organic eggplant, washed, peeled in horizontal stripes, and sliced into thin strips (if time permits, sprinkle the slices with salt and let them sit for 10 minutes to draw out excess moisture. Rinse thoroughly and pat dry for enhanced texture)

- 1 teaspoon freshly minced garlic

- 1 large organic red bell pepper, washed, seeded, and sliced into thin strips

- 2 large organic tomatoes, washed and diced

- 1 tablespoon organic tomato paste

- Sea salt and freshly ground black pepper, to taste

INSTRUCTIONS:

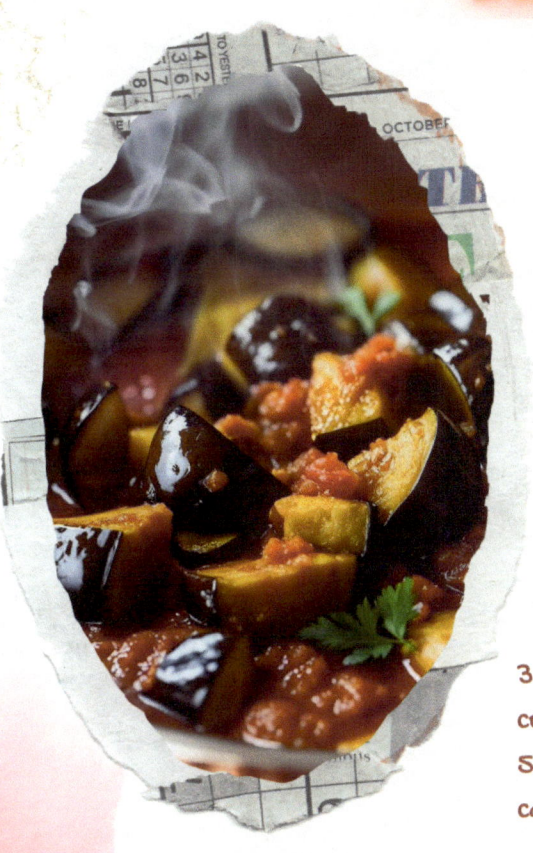

1. **Prepare the Eggplant:** Begin by heating a large stainless steel pot over medium heat for about two minutes. Once heated, add the extra-virgin olive oil, allowing it to warm for another minute.

2. **Sauté the Eggplant:** Carefully add the sliced eggplant to the pot, ensuring each piece is thoroughly coated in the oil. Cook the eggplant for about 5 minutes, stirring occasionally. Then, add the minced garlic and continue to sauté for an additional 2-3 minutes, allowing the flavors to meld and the eggplant to begin softening.

3. **Cook the Vegetables:** Reduce the heat to low, cover the pot, and let the eggplant cook gently for 5-7 minutes, until it becomes tender and slightly caramelized.

4. **Add the Remaining Ingredients:** Increase the heat back to medium-high and introduce the sliced red bell pepper, diced tomatoes, and tomato paste to the pot. Season with sea salt and freshly ground black pepper to taste. Stir the mixture vigorously for a couple of minutes to combine all the ingredients thoroughly.

5. **Simmer the Qorma:** Once combined, reduce the heat again, cover the pot with a lid, and allow it to simmer for 15 minutes. This will enable the vegetables to meld together and develop a rich flavor.

6. **Incorporate the Kidney Bean Qorma:** Gently fold in the prepared kidney bean qorma. (If you prefer a simpler dish, you can omit this step and enjoy the sautéed eggplant and vegetables on their own). Allow the mixture to cook for an additional 1-2 minutes to heat through.

7. **Serve:** Once done, taste and adjust the seasoning if necessary. This dish can be enjoyed hot, straight from the pot, or cooled and served as a refreshing side later on. Enjoy your vibrant and flavorful vegan creation!

The Hidden Path to Success: Baby Steps with Big Impact

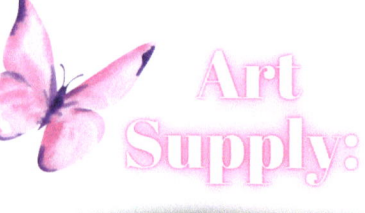

Imagine a secret staircase, tucked away behind an ordinary door. No grand leaps, no impossible bounds, just small, steady steps leading upward. The catch? Each step unlocks new strength, new confidence, and a glimpse of the extraordinary.

Step One: Break Through the Barrier

Dare to challenge yourself, but in a way that feels achievable. Progress isn't about reckless plunges, it's about stepping gently beyond your comfort zone, just enough to grow.

Step Two: The Power of 10 Minutes

Start with 10-15 minutes of movement daily. Not a grueling workout, not an overwhelming commitment, just simple momentum. Like the first footstep on the staircase, this small effort sets everything into motion.

Step Three: Watch the Snowball Roll

Small wins create momentum. One success fuels another, turning hesitation into habit. Before you know it, what once seemed impossible becomes second nature.

Step Four: Unlock the Hidden Reserves

Confidence rises with each milestone. Empowerment isn't just about achievement; it's about realizing you can keep pushing forward. Every step strengthens the next.

Final Step: The Transformation

With consistency, your staircase leads somewhere remarkable. You look back, surprised at how far you've come. The journey was never about a single giant leap, it was about mastering the art of small, purposeful steps.

Embrace the role of an artist as you navigate through your life's journey. Take a moment to truly observe the beauty that surrounds you, notice the vibrant colors that paint the landscape, the intricate details in everyday moments, and the unique patterns woven into the fabric of your experiences. Connect deeply with these elements, allowing them to inspire your thoughts and shape your perspective. Let your journey become a canvas, where each step reflects your creativity and appreciation for the world around you.

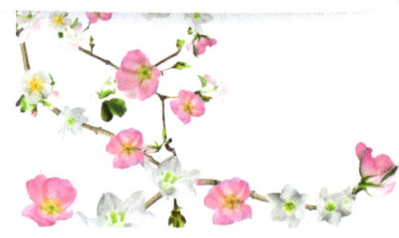

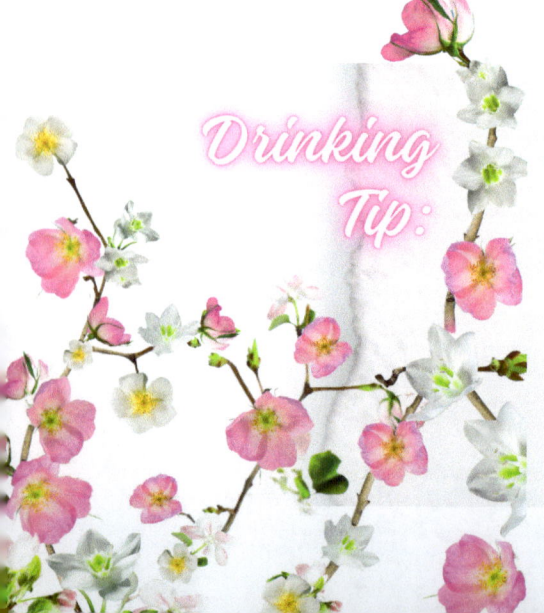

Drinking Tip:

Due to my struggle with anemia, I found myself running out of breath on the treadmill when I first started working out. I realized that staying hydrated was crucial, so I made sure to buy a high-quality water bottle to carry with me during workouts.

I stumbled upon a game-changer: tossing a dash of mineral salt into my water! It worked wonders on my breathlessness. Those snazzy electrolytes jazzed up my hydration and turbocharged my workout stamina!

One of the most challenging experiences I face is watching my beloved elderly relatives grapple with the effects of memory loss and, in some instances, Alzheimer's disease. Throughout my life, I have taken immense pride in these individuals who have navigated the complexities of existence with resilience, working tirelessly to create the best possible lives for their families and earning deep respect within their communities. However, witnessing their decline and the deterioration of their cognitive abilities raises profound questions in my mind: Was it truly worth it?

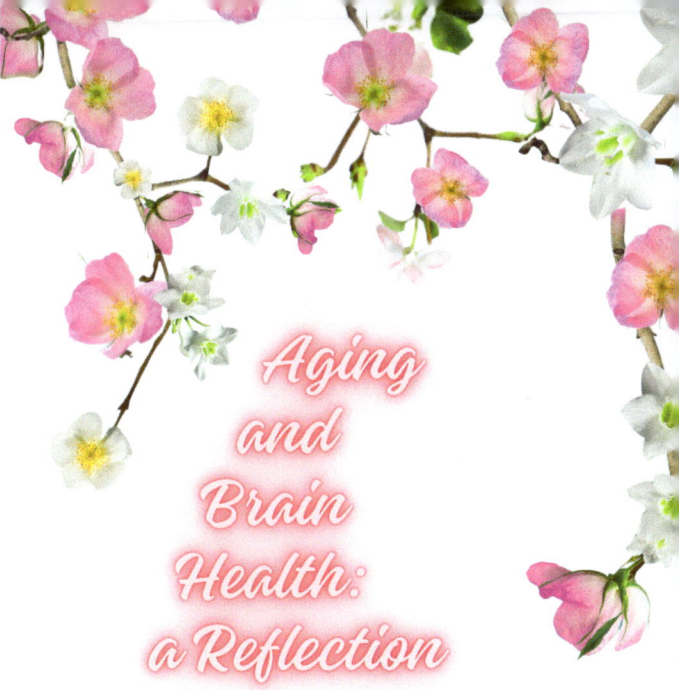

Aging and Brain Health: a Reflection

As I reflect on their journeys, I ponder whether they needed to choose the most difficult paths and race to what they believed was success in the shortest time possible. Did grabbing fast food on busy workdays justify the toll it took on their health? What about the sacrifices made, such as forgoing social engagements to fulfill the role of a great parent? Did the decision to skip the gym in order to put in extra hours at work ultimately pay off? And what of staying in a lackluster job just to meet financial obligations, did that really matter in the grand scheme of things? These thoughts lead me to consider whether rushing through life, with its myriad distractions, was truly the best approach.

As we navigate our daily lives, we often allow an overwhelming amount of noise and chaos to fill our minds. Instead of concentrating on attainable goals and making healthier life choices, we find ourselves entertaining thoughts that only add to our stress. Yet, I believe that if we shift our focus inward and commit to creating better plans, we can navigate life more effectively. Our brains are extraordinary organs that, if nurtured and given the opportunity, can significantly enhance our overall quality of life. Acknowledging this potential is essential for fostering a healthier relationship with ourselves and, ultimately, ensuring a more fulfilling existence as we age.

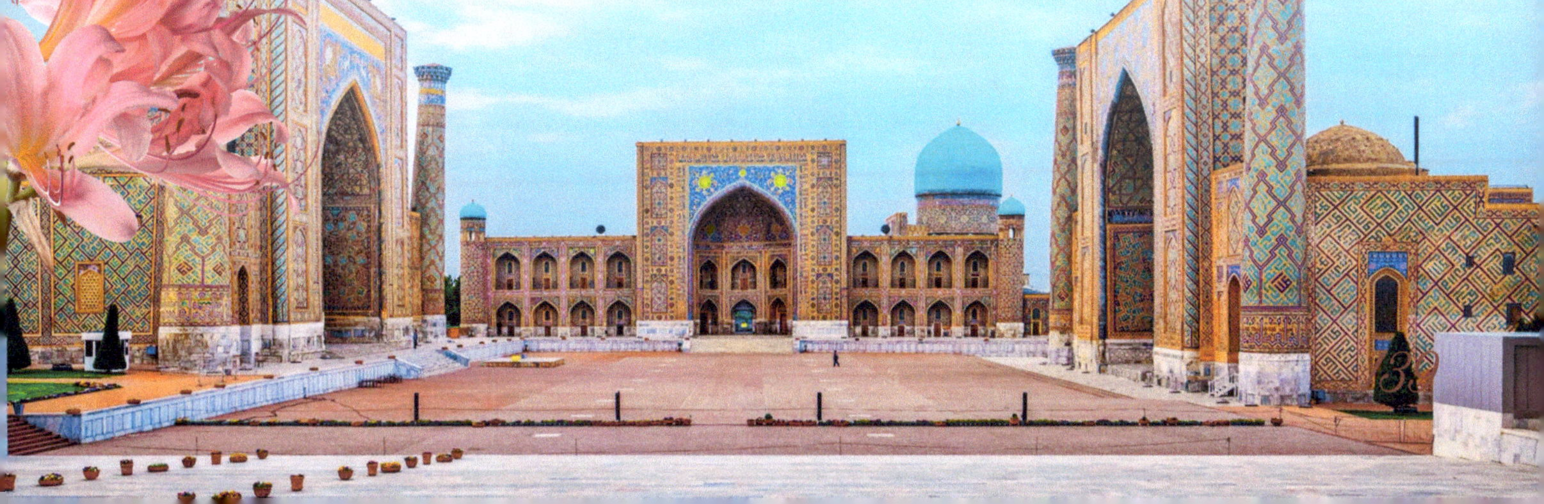

The Fastest Thing You Own

The brain is a living constellation, built from water, fat, protein, and minerals, yet capable of memory, myth, and transformation. It fires across 86 billion neurons at speeds up to 268 miles per hour. That's faster than a Formula 1 car. Faster than instinct. Faster than doubt.

Each thought, emotion, and breakthrough reshapes its circuitry in real time. This is neuroplasticity: the brain's ability to rewire itself, adapt, and evolve. You're not fixed. You're fluid. You're becoming.

It's 75% water, which means hydration isn't optional; it's sacred. This three-pound powerhouse consumes 20% of your body's energy, even when you're still. It's the hungriest, most demanding organ you have.

Even in sleep, it's working-regulating breath, processing dreams, solving problems. You rest. It recalibrates. You wake. It's already ahead of you.

Continue →

Brain Food: Tasty Treats for a Sharper Mind

Ever dream of unlocking your brain's full potential? Good news, your meals can be the key! With the right foods, you're not just eating; you're fueling focus, boosting memory, and setting the stage for long-term brain health.

Eggs: Nature's Cognitive Powerhouse

Think of eggs as tiny, golden orbs of wisdom. Packed with choline, they help sharpen memory and keep your mind firing on all cylinders. Plus, their high-quality protein and healthy fats make them a foundational staple for a brain-friendly diet.

Dark Chocolate: A Genius in Disguise

Indulgence meets intelligence in dark chocolate. Loaded with flavonoids, it enhances brain function, improves mood, and boosts concentration. Opt for the good stuff (70% cocoa or higher), and your brain will celebrate every bite.

Nuts: Little Brain-Shaped Wonders

Walnuts and almonds are rich in Omega-3s, which nourish the brain like a gentle wave of wisdom. Fun fact: Walnuts resemble tiny brains—is it nature's clever way of hinting at their brilliance? Before enjoying, try soaking them in filtered water for about 10 minutes. This unlocks even more nutrients and makes them easier to digest, because smart snacks should be gentle on the body, too.

Fresh, Local, and Organic: The Gold Standard

The secret to real nourishment? Quality. Prioritize organic, fresh, and local ingredients, and you'll do more than fuel your mind; you'll champion local farmers and nurture the planet. It's a win-win for your body and the world.

By filling your plate with these brain-boosting delights, you're investing in your sharpest, most vibrant self. After all, a healthy brain is the key to a happy, thriving life. So, why not savor every bite of wisdom?

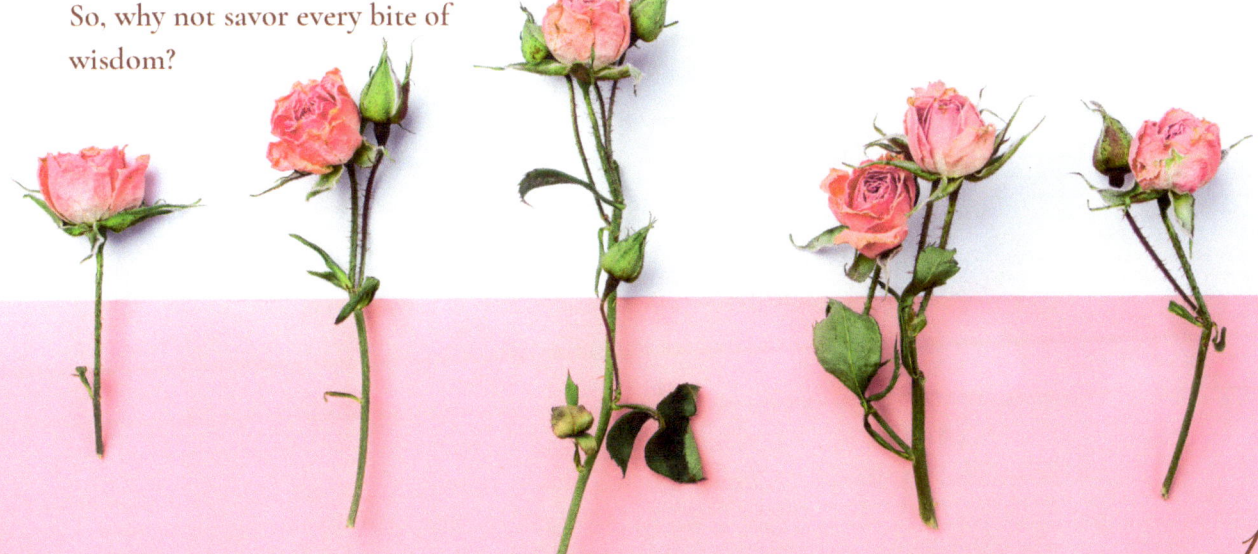

Twilight Spice Rice Paper Rolls

with Burnt Citrus Tahini & Pomegranate Dust

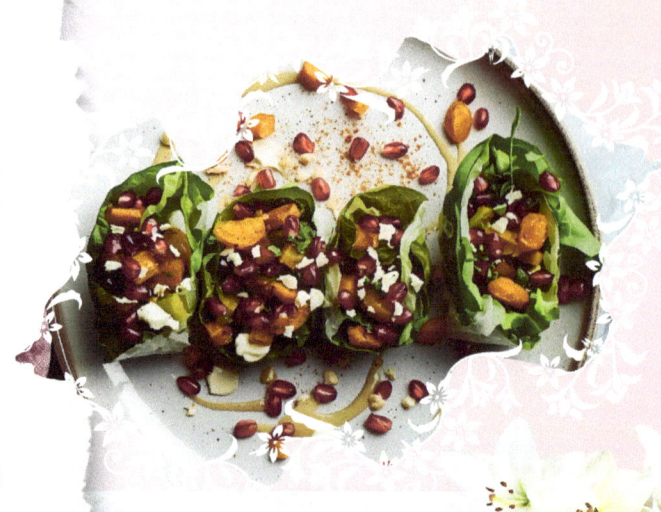

Filling Ingredients:

- Rice paper wrappers
- Filtered water
- Baby mustard greens or grape leaves (for bite and depth)
- Roasted eggplant strips (smoked over flame or pan-charred)
- Pickled turnip ribbons (for tang and crunch)
- Toasted cumin-roasted carrots (cut into matchsticks)

- Crushed pistachios or roasted chickpeas
- Fresh mint and tarragon
- Black seeds (kalonji)
- Dried barberries or pomegranate arils
- Optional: slivers of dried apricot soaked in saffron water

To Assemble:

Soften rice paper in warm water. Layer greens first, then eggplant, turnip, carrots, and crunch. Add herbs, seeds, and fruit. Roll tightly. Serve with burnt citrus tahini, dusted with pomegranate.

Burnt Citrus Tahini Sauce

This isn't your average drizzle; it's a smoky, sour, bitter-sweet balm.

Ingredients:

- 2 tbsp tahini
- Juice of ½ charred orange (grill or pan-sear the cut side)
- Splash of lemon juice
- 1 tsp pomegranate molasses
- Pinch of ground coriander
- Sea salt to taste
- Ice-cold water to thin
- Optional: crushed dried rose petals or sumac for garnish

Instructions:

- Whisk tahini with burnt orange juice, lemon, molasses, and coriander.
- Add cold water slowly until silky.
- Taste for balance; this sauce should feel like dusk: smoky, sour, and slightly floral.
- Garnish with rose petals or sumac if serving in a bowl.

Zaatar-Dusted Cucumber Boats

with Date-Lime Labneh
(a cooling snack for clarity and calm)

Ingredients:

- Persian cucumbers, halved lengthwise and hollowed slightly
- Labneh or thick yogurt
- Chopped medjool dates
- Fresh lime zest
- Zaatar
- Crushed pistachios
- Sea salt

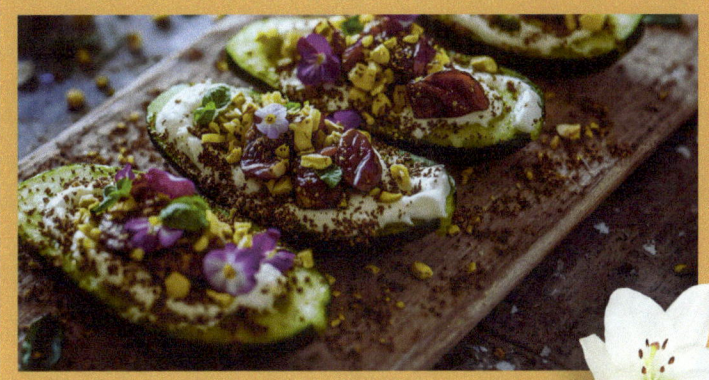

Assembly:

1. Mix labneh with chopped dates and lime zest until creamy.
2. Spoon into cucumber boats.
3. Dust with zaatar, pistachios, and a pinch of sea salt.
4. Chill briefly before serving.

Why it heals:

Crunch cools the nerves.
Zaatar sharpens the mind.
Dates soften the heart.
And lime reminds you, bitterness can be bright.

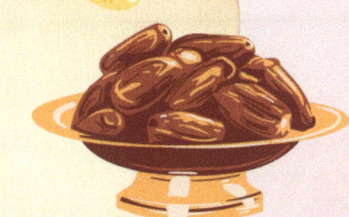

These recipes don't just teach you to cook, they teach you to continue. To turn 'too little' into 'just enough.' To stretch a story instead of ending it. To look into a fridge and see possibility, not limitation. And maybe, just maybe, to trust that nourishment often comes in the reworking, not the start.

Listen to Your Body:

Pause for a second. Not the polite kind of pause, but the kind where you actually notice yourself—the weight of your feet on the floor, the rhythm of your breath, the quiet hum of being alive. Feels kind of wild, right? Because here's the truth: most of us spend our days bending and twisting ourselves to fit into someone else's idea of who we should be. We chase deadlines, scroll endlessly, smile when we're tired, and forget the one thing that never forgets us; our bodies.

And oh, what a treasure they are. Your body is not just a shell you drag around; it's a 24/7 miracle machine. Your heart? It's been beating since before you were born, never once asking for a break. Your lungs? They've been inflating and deflating like the most loyal accordion, keeping you alive while you sleep, dream, and binge-watch shows. Your digestive system? It's basically a chemistry lab, breaking down food into fuel with the precision of a master alchemist.

But here's the part that feels like opening a secret map: your body talks to you. Constantly. That tightness in your shoulders? A flare of stress. That sudden craving for something salty? A whisper about minerals. That restless energy at midnight? A nudge that your mind and body are out of sync. These aren't random quirks; they're clues, little golden coins scattered along the path to understanding yourself.

The problem is, we've been trained to ignore them. We drown fatigue in coffee, silence hunger with distraction, push through pain because "there's no time." And in doing so, we miss the treasure chest sitting right in front of us.

So what if you flipped the script? What if you treated your body like the most fascinating book you'll ever read, one where every ache, sigh, and spark of energy is a sentence worth decoding? Suddenly, life feels less like a grind and more like an adventure. You're not just existing, you're discovering.

Because here's the secret: your body isn't against you. It's your fiercest ally, your built-in compass, your most loyal friend. And the moment you start listening-really listening-you unlock a kind of wisdom that no app, no trend, no outside voice can give you.

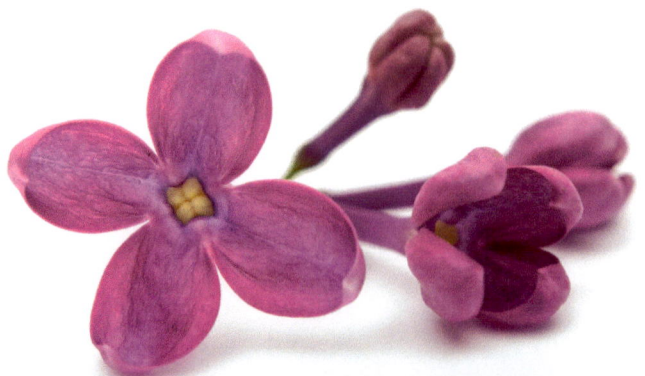

144

The Body's Secret Language: Listening to the Messages Beneath the Skin:

And this idea, that the body is more than muscle and bone, more than a machine to be pushed or ignored, isn't just a modern revelation. Across centuries, cultures have looked at the body as a mirror of the mind and spirit, a living manuscript where emotions, struggles, and triumphs leave their mark. What we're rediscovering today through science is something humanity has always known: the body speaks, and every civilization has tried to learn its language.

In ancient Greece, philosophers debated the soul's connection to the body, was it merely a vessel, or were the two inseparable? Meanwhile, traditional Chinese medicine mapped emotions onto organs, believing that frustration could lodge itself in the liver, grief in the lungs, and suppressed expression in the throat. Ayurveda saw energy centers, chakras, as key to both emotional and physical well-being. Across cultures, the idea remained the same: emotions don't just live in the mind; they leave their mark on the body.

Even medieval thought wrestled with this relationship, viewing the body as a site of spiritual and emotional struggle. But as time marched on, Western thinking increasingly separated mind and body, treating them as distinct entities rather than interconnected forces. Only now, as neuroscience advances, is science confirming what ancient wisdom long suspected; stress weakens immunity, anxiety tightens muscles, trauma lingers in the body long after the mind moves on.

So when your knees ache or your neck stiffens, it's not just wear and tear, it might be your body speaking in an ancient language, one that has echoed through time. By listening, reflecting, and understanding these signals, we reconnect with a wisdom that has shaped human experience for millennia.

Hormone Balance: a Personal Journey

Hormones shape the rhythm of our lives, quietly orchestrating the forces that lift us up or pull us down. They dictate how effortlessly we rise in the morning, how deeply we laugh, how much energy pulses through our veins. When balanced, they infuse every moment with vitality, fueling ambition, clarity, and an innate joy for simply being. But when thrown into chaos, they leave ripples across the mind and body, whispering through exhaustion, reshaping emotions, and distorting the familiar into something unrecognizable.

I have felt this unraveling, the slow, quiet shift where something no longer feels right, though you can't quite name it. It came not as a single moment but as an accumulation, woven into the changes that altered my life's rhythm. A new city, a new job, marriage, three pillars that should have marked the foundation of growth, yet instead left me adrift in uncertainty. The routines around me belonged to others, the expectations unfamiliar, and in my eagerness to blend in, I lost the vibrant pulse of my own identity.

I was young, searching for stability in the reflection of others, colleagues, friends, family, all the while unknowingly surrendering pieces of myself. In my effort to be seen, I had dimmed the very essence that made me feel alive. Slowly, I found myself retreating into an emotional fog, where the weight of unspoken discomfort pressed against my chest, where joy felt distant and exhaustion felt endless.

Hormonal imbalance was not just a medical condition, it was a conversation, a message from my body telling me that something had been lost. And in the act of listening, of slowing down, of reclaiming my own rhythm, I began to restore balance, not just within my body, but within my life.

I did not vanish from the world, I faded. Slowly, quietly, like ink dissolving into water. It was not rejection that pushed me inward, nor was it isolation. It was the quiet erosion of my own voice, the slow surrender of my essence to the expectations of others. And in that silence, something within me began to unravel.

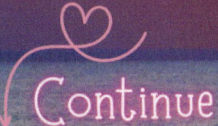

Continue

At first, it was subtle. A heaviness in my limbs, a dullness in my thoughts, a quiet exhaustion that settled into my bones. The days blurred, each one carrying the same weight, the same absence of joy. I moved through life as if watching from a distance, detached from the pulse of my own existence. My body, once vibrant and alive, had become a stranger to me.

The journey back was not a single moment of revelation; it was a slow, deliberate return. It required me to sift through the layers of expectation, to unearth the pieces of myself I had buried in my effort to belong. I had to ask the questions I had long avoided: Who was I beneath the roles I had adopted? What did I truly desire, beyond the approval of others? The answers did not come all at once, but in fragments, small, luminous truths that I gathered like scattered stars.

I reclaimed myself in the simplest of ways. I sought out the things that once made me feel alive, the books that stirred my imagination, the music that made my heart race, the quiet moments where I could simply exist without explanation. I let go of the need to mold myself into someone else's vision, choosing instead to stand fully in my own.

And slowly, the balance returned. Not just in my body, but in my spirit. The weight lifted, the fog cleared, and I felt the quiet certainty of something I had nearly forgotten: I was whole, I was enough, and I was free.

Hormonal
balance, I realized,
was never just about
biology. It was about alignment,
about living in harmony with oneself,
about honoring the rhythms that are uniquely ours.
It was about listening to the whispers of the body, the quiet
urgings of the soul, and allowing them to guide us back to where we belong.

DITCH THE FAKE, EMBRACE THE REAL: WHY GRASS-FED MEAT IS THE ULTIMATE UPGRADE

If you enjoy eating meat, choose wisely, because every bite carries a story. Grass-fed options from local farms aren't just about nutrition; they are about integrity, about honoring the natural rhythm of life itself. These farms prioritize respect, allowing animals to roam freely, graze on untouched pastures, and live without the burden of synthetic hormones. It's a return to what food was always meant to be—pure, unaltered, deeply nourishing.

When you choose grass-fed, you are not simply selecting a healthier option, you are aligning with something greater. You are supporting a world where animals live as they were meant to, breathing fresh air, moving with ease, thriving in nature rather than being confined to sterile feedlots. Their lives are fuller, their bodies stronger, and in turn, the nourishment they offer is more potent, rich in omega-3s, antioxidants, and essential vitamins that fuel you exactly as nature intended.

This is more than a meal. It is a movement, a ripple of choice that extends beyond the plate, shaping a food system that values compassion over convenience, quality over mass production. And when you sit down to eat, knowing that what's before you came from a place of care, respect, and ethical stewardship, it transforms the experience entirely. It becomes sustenance with a soul, nourishment with a purpose.

So, if you are ready to feed your body while honoring the earth, choose grass-fed. Choose food that carries the richness of nature, the purity of tradition, and the promise of a better way forward.

Cayenne:

Harness the potent benefits of cayenne pepper, known for its ability to significantly enhance your immune system, making it an excellent ally in fighting off illnesses. This spicy sidekick boosts circulation, paving the way for a heart-healthy journey and first-class nutrient delivery throughout your body. Plus, cayenne spices things up by battling against candida overgrowth, restoring harmony in your gut's bustling metropolis.

In addition to these advantages, cayenne supports effective detoxification processes, aiding your body in flushing out harmful toxins and impurities. It also plays a valuable role in weight management, as it may help boost metabolism and increase fat burning. Enrich your health with this vitamin A-rich powerhouse and enjoy its multiple wellness benefits.

Cilantro:

My mom always had a strong preference for garnishing food with fresh cilantro, and I never quite shared her enthusiasm for it! No matter how much effort I put into creating visually stunning dishes topped with spring flowers, they consistently fell short in my mother's eyes due to the absence of cilantro. I recently came across a medical report stating that cilantro can help cleanse and detoxify the liver by removing heavy metals. Accumulation of heavy metals in the liver can potentially interfere with gut health, and I know me; my liver is my treasure, so finally, I accepted cilantro in my diet! Not as garnish, in my juicer with mint leaves, apples, and ginger. Cilantro contains compounds that may aid in the chelation (removal) of heavy metals from the body, contributing to overall liver health and potentially benefiting gut health as well.

Also, it helps reverse candida overgrowth, boosts immunity with its rich nutrient content, reduces inflammation thanks to its anti-inflammatory properties, and supports bone health with its high levels of vitamin K and calcium.

So garnish on, or even better, juice on!

Everglow

My mother-in-law was known for her radiant complexion, the kind of glow that seemed to come from both inside and out. She had her rituals - a thin layer of yogurt smoothed across her face before gatherings, vegetable peels resting cool beneath her eyes. At first, I thought of it as vanity, a small performance before stepping into the world. But over time, I began to see it differently: as armor, as preparation, as a way of softening whatever might come.

Yogurt, after all, is more than a mask. Its lactic acid gently dissolves what no longer serves the skin, revealing something brighter beneath. It soothes, it balances, it restores. Watching her, I realized that her true glow wasn't just the result of enzymes or probiotics - it was her refusal to let life's harsher elements etch themselves too deeply. She carried positivity like a shield, even when the air around her was less than kind.

I sometimes wondered if the yogurt was her quiet metaphor: a reminder that even when the world feels sharp, there are ways to protect, to renew, to keep something luminous alive. That glow was not effortless. It was chosen, cultivated, tended.

And that is what I carry with me now. Not just the recipe for smoother skin, but the lesson that renewal is possible - that even in environments that can be demanding, even in roles that press heavy on the spirit, there are ways to keep your light intact. Her glow was never only on her face. It was in her resilience, her joy, her insistence on beauty where others might have surrendered.

Healthy Nibbles

Pistachios:

Pistachios remind me of moments that ask nothing but presence. The slow crack of the shell, the soft green reveal, the way they feel earthy and elegant all at once.

They're rich in healthy fats and antioxidants that support brain health, not loudly, but steadily. Their low glycemic index makes them a gentle companion for blood sugar balance, especially for those navigating diabetes with care. And with protein and fiber, they offer satiety without heaviness.

There's Vitamin B6, quietly orchestrating neurotransmitters and metabolism. And minerals, copper, manganese, phosphorus, thiamin, woven in like threads of resilience.

I don't eat pistachios for the science. I eat them because they feel like a pause. A small, nourishing act that reminds me I'm worth tending to.

Pumpkin seeds:

I've always had a soft spot for pumpkin seeds. It started with the simple joy of roasting them after carving pumpkins, warm, nutty, and just the right kind of crunch. But over time, I realized they're more than just a nostalgic snack. These little seeds are inflammation-fighters, focus-boosters, and immune supporters. They even lend a hand with healthy weight management.

Nutritionally, they're stacked: rich in magnesium, manganese, and phosphorus, plus a solid dose of iron, protein, and zinc.

They're the kind of everyday superfood that doesn't need to shout. Just a handful, and you're doing something kind for your body, without making a big production of it.

The Power of Us:
Strength Through Community

We were never meant to stand alone.
From the moment we take our first breath, we
belong to something greater than just ourselves. The people we
surround ourselves with define our resilience, our success, our ability
to thrive.
Long ago, a father nearing the end of his life called
his children to his side. He handed them a bundle of
sticks and asked
each to break it. One by one, they tried, but no
matter how strong they were, the bundle held firm. Then, he untied
it and gave them a single stick each. This time, they snapped
effortlessly.

Alone, we are fragile. Together, we are unbreakable.
This is the essence of community, the power of unity, the strength in numbers, the
force of people standing side by side. The greatest achievements in history were
never the work of just one, they were the result of shared vision, collective effort,
and unwavering support.
When we stand with others, we push past limitations. Teams conquer challenges that
individuals cannot. Shared wisdom accelerates growth. A trusted network provides
the resilience needed to weather life's storms.

- Want success? Find your people.
- Want strength? Lean on your allies.
- Want purpose? Build something bigger than yourself.

Because life moves in waves, sometimes calm, sometimes wild. But with the right community, you always have steady ground.

Even science confirms it; relationships impact every part of our well-being. Strong connections boost mental health, sharpen focus, even increase lifespan. Loneliness drains us, but belonging fortifies. The bonds we choose shape our future.

And here's the core truth: one for all, all for one. A thriving community lifts everyone within it. When you invest in those around you, their strength becomes your strength, their victories your victories. The more we support, uplift, and move together, the greater we all become.

So, choose wisely, invest deeply, and stand with those who stand with you. Because just like that bundle of sticks, alone we break, together, we endure.

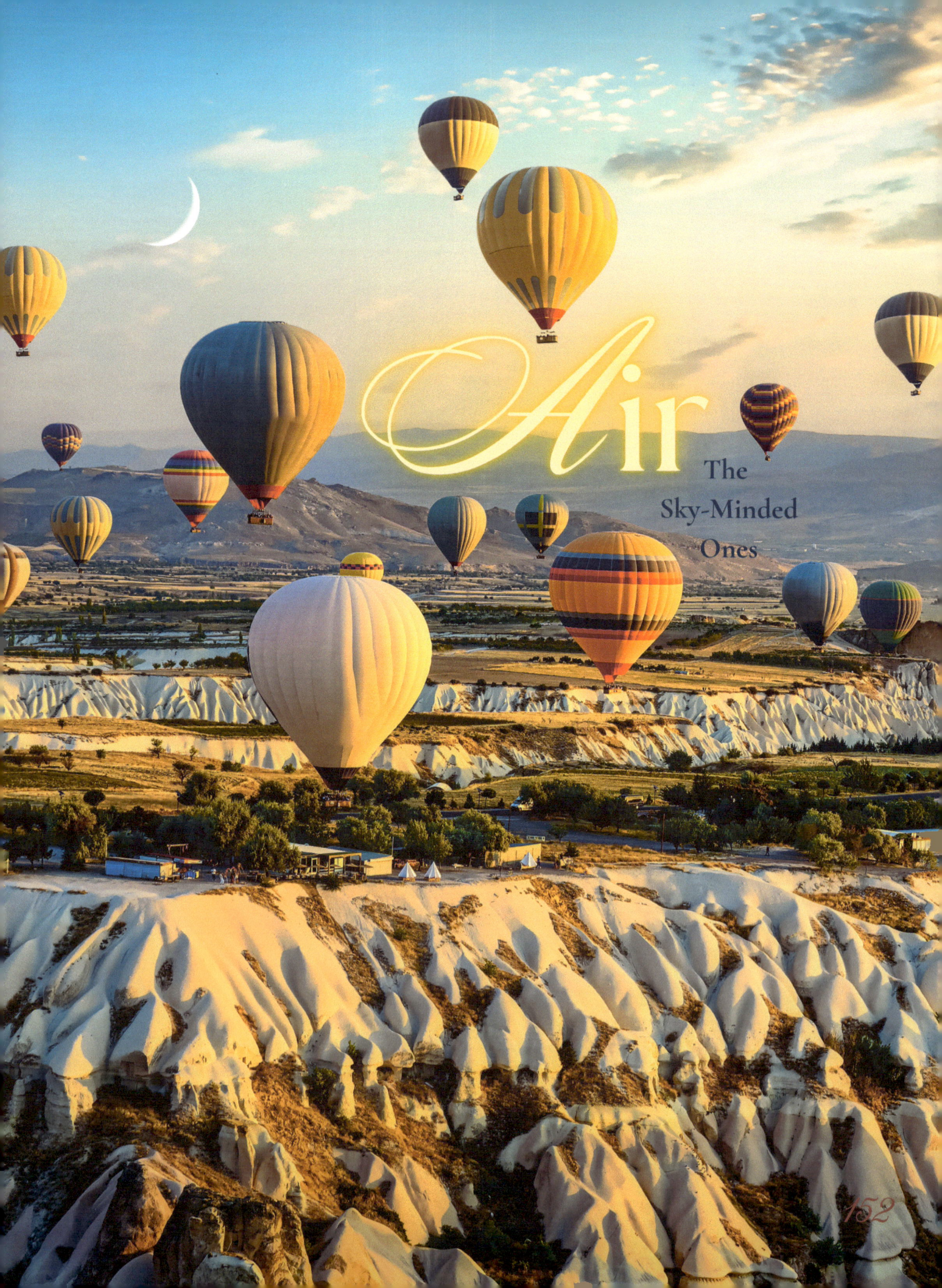

Air

The
Sky-Minded
Ones

Air is the element of motion, of mind, of breath. It does not ask permission—it moves. It thinks. It speaks. It questions. It is the restless pulse behind every idea, the invisible force that lifts words into meaning and meaning into change.

To be an air soul is to live in the realm of thought. These are the ones who speak in spirals, who chase clarity like wind chases open fields. They are brilliant, quick, and endlessly curious. They connect dots others don't see. They build bridges with language, sketch futures with questions, and stir revolutions in quiet rooms.
But air does not settle. It resists stillness. It floats above the body, above emotion, above the moment. It can scatter. It can forget to land.

Air types often feel most alive in conversation, in ideation, in the electric hum of possibility. They thrive on novelty, perspective, and the freedom to roam mentally and spiritually. But without grounding, they can become untethered-lost in abstraction, disconnected from their own needs, from the earth beneath them.

They need anchors. Not cages. Not rules. But rituals. Relationships. Rhythms. They need the weight of presence to balance their flight. A walk in silence. A meal cooked slowly. A friend who listens without trying to fix. A notebook that catches the whirlwind before it disappears.

Air is not weak. It is not flaky. It is the element of transformation through thought. But even the sky needs a horizon. Even the wind needs trees to shape its song.
To honor air is to honor the thinkers, the communicators, the ones who carry the future in their breath. And to care for them is to remind them: you are allowed to land. You are allowed to feel. You are allowed to be held.
Let your thoughts fly. But let your soul rest.

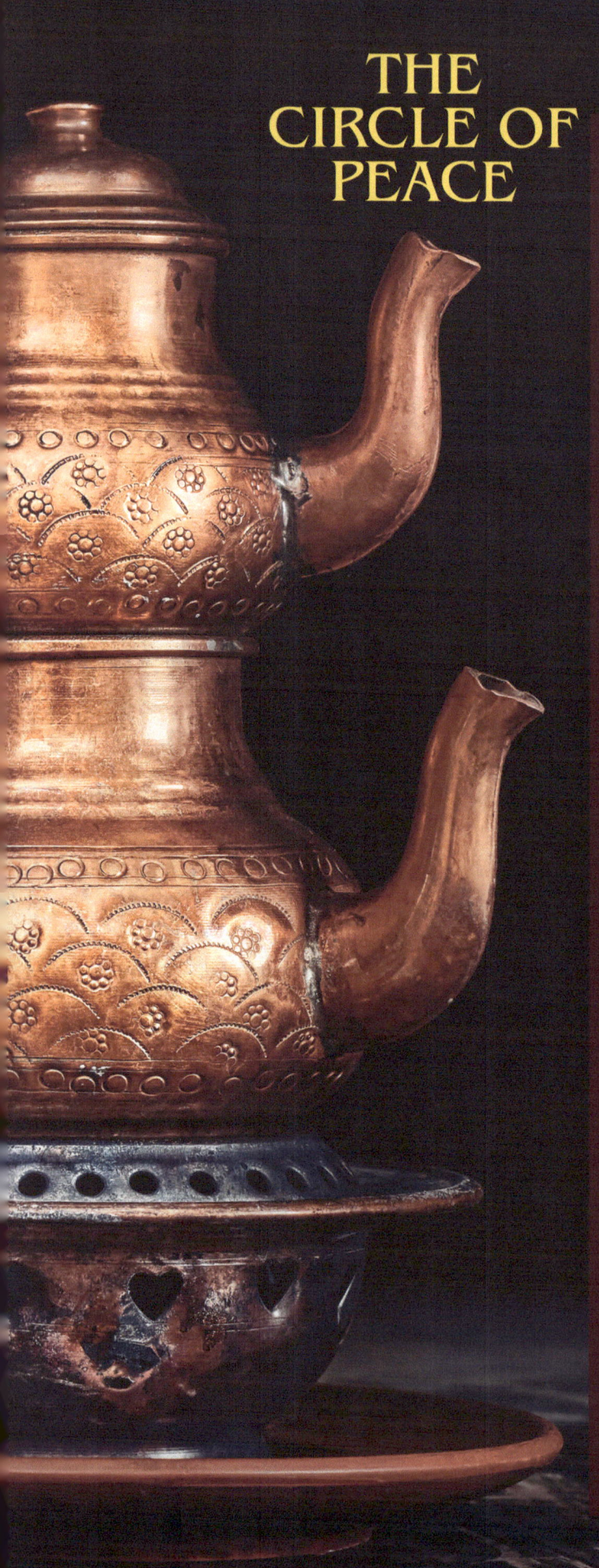

THE CIRCLE OF PEACE

To beautify your inner world is to relinquish what was never yours to hold. Not every whisper belongs in your ear. Not every headline deserves a home in your heart.

Imagine your mind as a circle, small, sacred, and sufficient. Within it: your breath, your prayers, your people. Outside it: the noise. The less you know of what lies beyond, the more you can feel what lives within. Peace is not found in knowing everything. It is found in knowing what to forget. Once, the world moved slower. A letter took weeks. A rumor arrived softened by time. News was not a flood, it was a story, told over tea, shaped by memory and mercy. There was space to feel before reacting. Space to live before labeling.

Now, we are flooded. We know too much, too fast. A stranger's grief becomes our own. A scandal in a city we've never seen steals our sleep. We scroll through suffering, mistaking awareness for wisdom. But wisdom is selective. It knows when to turn away.

I once met a woman who lived in the mountains, no phone, no television. She knew the names of birds, the moods of clouds, the scent of rain before it fell. Her world was small, but her soul was vast. "I don't need to know everything," she said, "just enough to love what's mine."

Her daughter, a journalist, visited once a year. She brought stories, wars, elections, celebrity divorces. The mother listened, then asked, "But how is your heart?" The daughter wept. No one had asked her that in months.

So let your circle be small. Let your knowing be gentle. Let your peace be protected. The world will keep spinning. You don't have to hold it all.

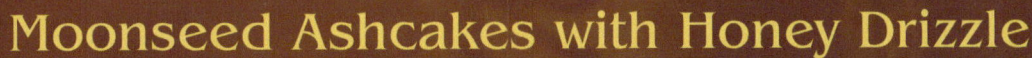

Moonseed Ashcakes with Honey Drizzle

A humble, rustic bread inspired by ancient cooking, made for calm moments and simple pleasures.

Why it's unique

This recipe combines an old-fashioned fire-cooking method (ashcakes) with a creative ingredient (moonseed flour) symbolizing something rare and thoughtful. You can substitute with buckwheat flour and black sesame for a nutty, wholesome flavor. The honey drizzle adds a gentle sweetness to balance the bread's earthy notes.

Ingredients: (makes 4 small ashcakes)

- 1 cup moonseed flour (or substitute: finely ground buckwheat and crushed black sesame seeds)
- ½ tsp salt
- 1 tsp crushed fennel seeds (for a subtle, warm aroma)
- ½ tsp dried mint (optional, for freshness)
- ½ cup warm water
- 1 tbsp olive oil or melted ghee
- Optional: 1 tsp edible charcoal powder (for color and subtle smokiness)

Honey Drizzle:

- 2 tbsp raw honey
- 1 drop rosewater (optional)
- Pinch of saffron or turmeric (optional, for color and gentle flavor)

Instructions:

1. In a bowl, combine the dry ingredients. Add warm water and oil, mixing gently until a soft dough forms.
2. Shape the dough into small, flat rounds, about the size of your palm.
3. Heat a cast-iron pan or heavy skillet over medium heat. Cook the rounds directly on the dry pan until both sides are firm and lightly browned, about 4-5 minutes per side.
4. While the ashcakes are cooking, gently warm the honey and stir in rosewater and saffron or turmeric if using.
5. Drizzle the honey over the warm ashcakes before serving.

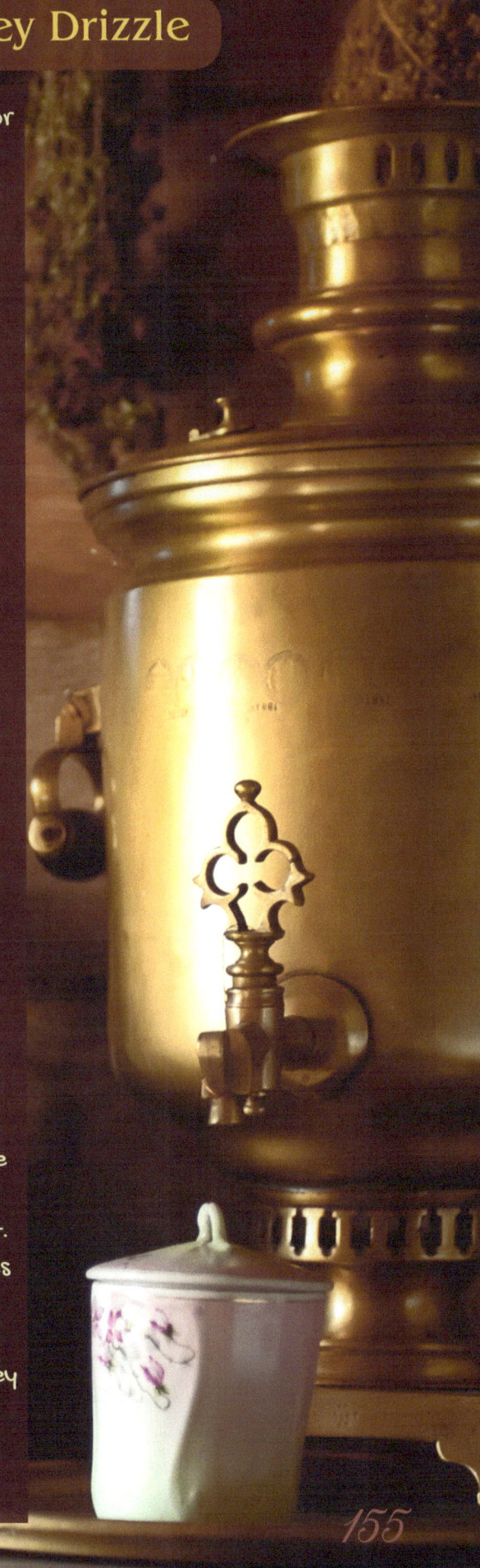

155

HOME IMPROVMENT

What does home mean to an individual? A home transcends the notion of a mere physical structure; it serves as a cherished sanctuary that both shelters our aspirations and nurtures our innermost selves. It is the first sight that greets us when we awaken each morning, wrapping us in a comforting embrace as we prepare to embark on a new day filled with possibilities. Similarly, it is the last vision we hold before surrendering to sleep, imparting a profound sense of security and belonging that is essential to our well-being.

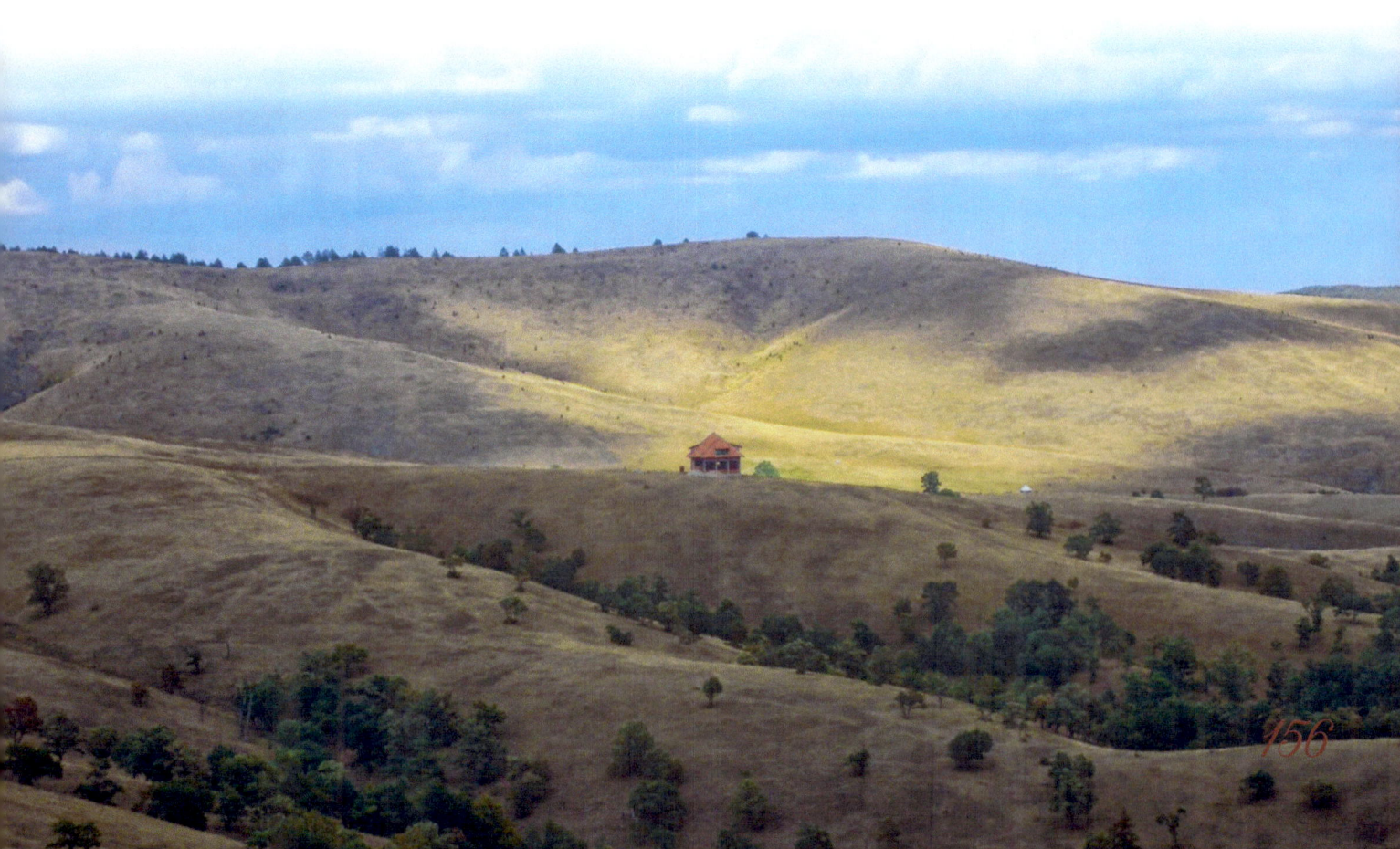

A home is not only a structure, not just walls and a roof; it is the heart of our existence, the stage upon which our lives unfold. It absorbs our energy, amplifies our spirit, and extends our very essence into every corner. It is a reflection, a mirror of who we are, woven with the threads of our experiences, dreams, and silent aspirations.

And science agrees, our environment directly shapes our mental and physical well-being. Studies show that cluttered spaces can elevate stress hormones, while intentional, well-organized surroundings encourage mental clarity, lower cortisol levels, and even enhance creativity. Simply put: the state of your home influences the state of your mind.

Every detail, every carefully chosen piece of decor carries meaning, whispering our personalities into space. The photographs lining the walls, the worn edges of a favorite book, the way sunlight spills onto the floors in the quiet moments of morning, these are not just objects; they are extensions of us.

But the soul of a home is shaped not by possessions alone, but by the energy within it. The atmosphere we cultivate is a reflection of our inner world. A chaotic mind leads to cluttered spaces; unresolved emotions manifest in the disorder that unsettles the very sanctuary meant to bring us peace.

Our ancestors understood this deeply; their homes were not simply places to sleep, but sacred spaces where life, tradition, and human connection thrived. Ancient cultures mastered the art of harmonizing their environment, recognizing that what surrounds us shapes us. Feng Shui, for example, is rooted in optimizing energy flow within a home to enhance well-being, while minimalism teaches that simplicity brings mental freedom.

A home should restore, should breathe, should uplift. It should be a sanctuary, not just in design, but in feeling, a place where the weight of the outside world dissolves, where tranquility is not merely a concept but a presence.

Recognizing this deep connection between our surroundings and our state of mind allows us to shape our homes with intention, not just filling them with beauty, but infusing them with serenity, balance, and renewal. When we nurture both the physical and emotional essence of our space, we create more than a home; we create a refuge, a sanctuary that sustains us.

And so, the journey begins, not in grand gestures, but in the smallest details. In the way we arrange, the way we care, the way we choose to be present within the space that holds our lives.

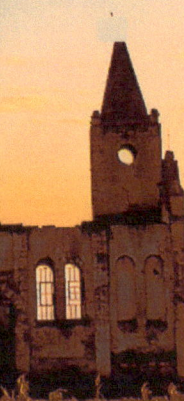

HOUSE PROUD TIPS: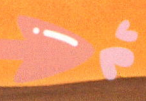

1. Deeeeeeclutter:

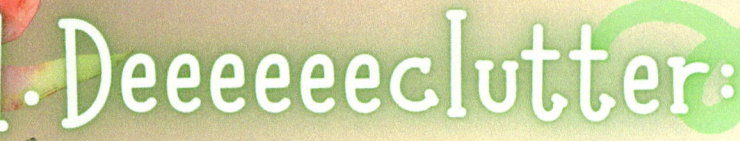

I love collecting things and holding onto items with sentimental value. For example, I still have some shirts from my 20s that I hope to fit into again one day. Additionally, I have a habit of keeping empty boxes and pretty bags because I find them useful for storage and gifting. During the fall season, my living space is adorned with all kinds of pumpkins, adding a festive touch to the decor. As for other items, I have a collection of old toys, clothes that no one wears in the house, and a few mismatched pieces of dishes that used to be part of a set. However, I've come to realize that I DON'T NEED THEM! These things no longer serve a purpose in my life.! When an object hasn't been utilized in my household in the past 12 months, it's time to find new homes for it, donate or sell, period.

My aunt's advice was more than just a household tip; it was a philosophy, a quiet truth about the energy we invite into our lives. She taught me that the space beneath the bed should remain clear, and the top of the clothes cabinet should be free of clutter, because disorder has a way of holding onto stagnant energy. At the time, it seemed like a simple rule, but as I grew older, I began to understand its deeper significance.

Clutter is not just physical, it is emotional, mental, even spiritual. A crowded space can weigh on the mind, creating a sense of heaviness, distraction, and unease. When objects pile up, they don't just take up room; they hold onto energy, trapping us in cycles of procrastination, stress, and even fatigue. Clearing these spaces is more than tidying, it is an act of renewal, a way to invite clarity, movement, and fresh energy into our lives.

There is something profoundly freeing about an open space, about knowing that beneath your bed, there is nothing lurking, no forgotten items gathering dust, no stagnant energy lingering in the shadows. And when the tops of cabinets remain clear, the room breathes easier, the air feels lighter, and the mind follows suit. It is a small act, yet its impact is undeniable.

I hold my aunt's words close, not just as advice, but as a quiet ritual—a way to honor the flow of energy, to create space for new beginnings, and to ensure that the places I call home remain not just organized, but alive with possibility.

2. Paint:

Paint the walls if possible; select a color that speaks to you and brings a sense of joy and happiness to your soul. It's truly remarkable how colors can have a strong impact on our emotions and overall mood.

3. House Plants:

Consider getting indoor plants, as they can significantly improve air quality by removing toxins and releasing oxygen. Moreover, they can add a refreshing and natural touch to any room, enhancing its aesthetic appeal. Additionally, indoor plants have been shown to have a positive impact on mental well-being by boosting mood, reducing stress, and improving concentration. Lastly, and the best part, indoor plants are natural air purifiers.

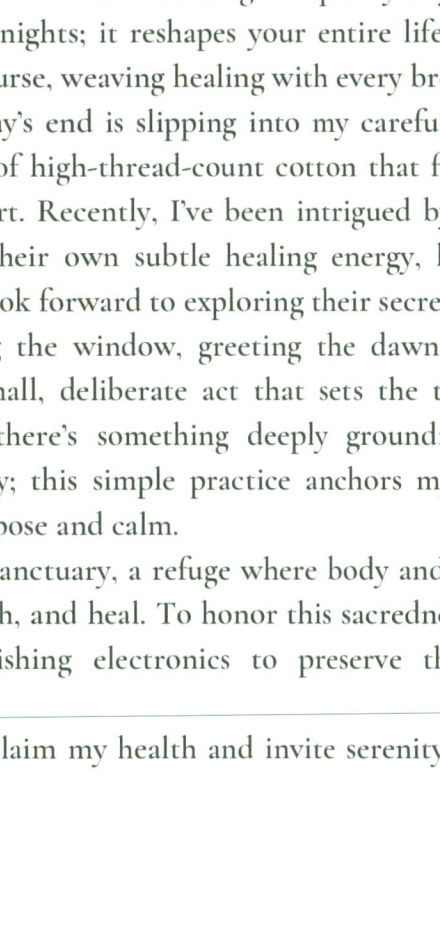

4. Pay Extra Attention to The Bedroom:

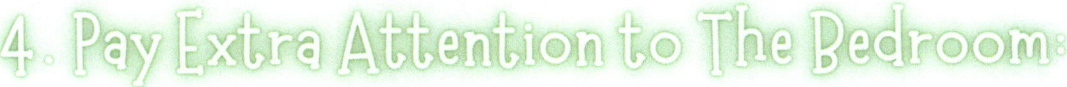

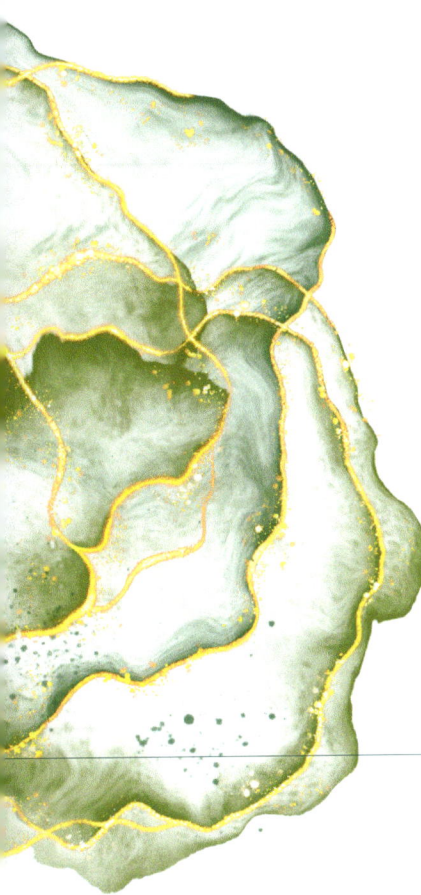

The bedroom is where the magic quietly unfolds, the sacred space where rest transforms into renewal. Elevating the quality of your sleep doesn't just change your nights; it reshapes your entire life. Sleep is, after all, nature's gentle nurse, weaving healing with every breath.

My favorite custom at day's end is slipping into my carefully chosen sheets; the soft embrace of high-thread-count cotton that feels like a tender promise of comfort. Recently, I've been intrigued by the idea that linen sheets carry their own subtle healing energy, hinting at overnight restoration. I look forward to exploring their secrets.

I arrange my bed facing the window, greeting the dawn with the vastness of the sky, a small, deliberate act that sets the tone for a hopeful morning. And there's something deeply grounding about making the bed each day; this simple practice anchors my essence, infusing the day with purpose and calm.

Truly, the bedroom is a sanctuary, a refuge where body and soul find space to breathe, replenish, and heal. To honor this sacredness, I keep technology at bay, banishing electronics to preserve the room's tranquil embrace.

In this quiet refuge, I reclaim my health and invite serenity to settle, night after night.

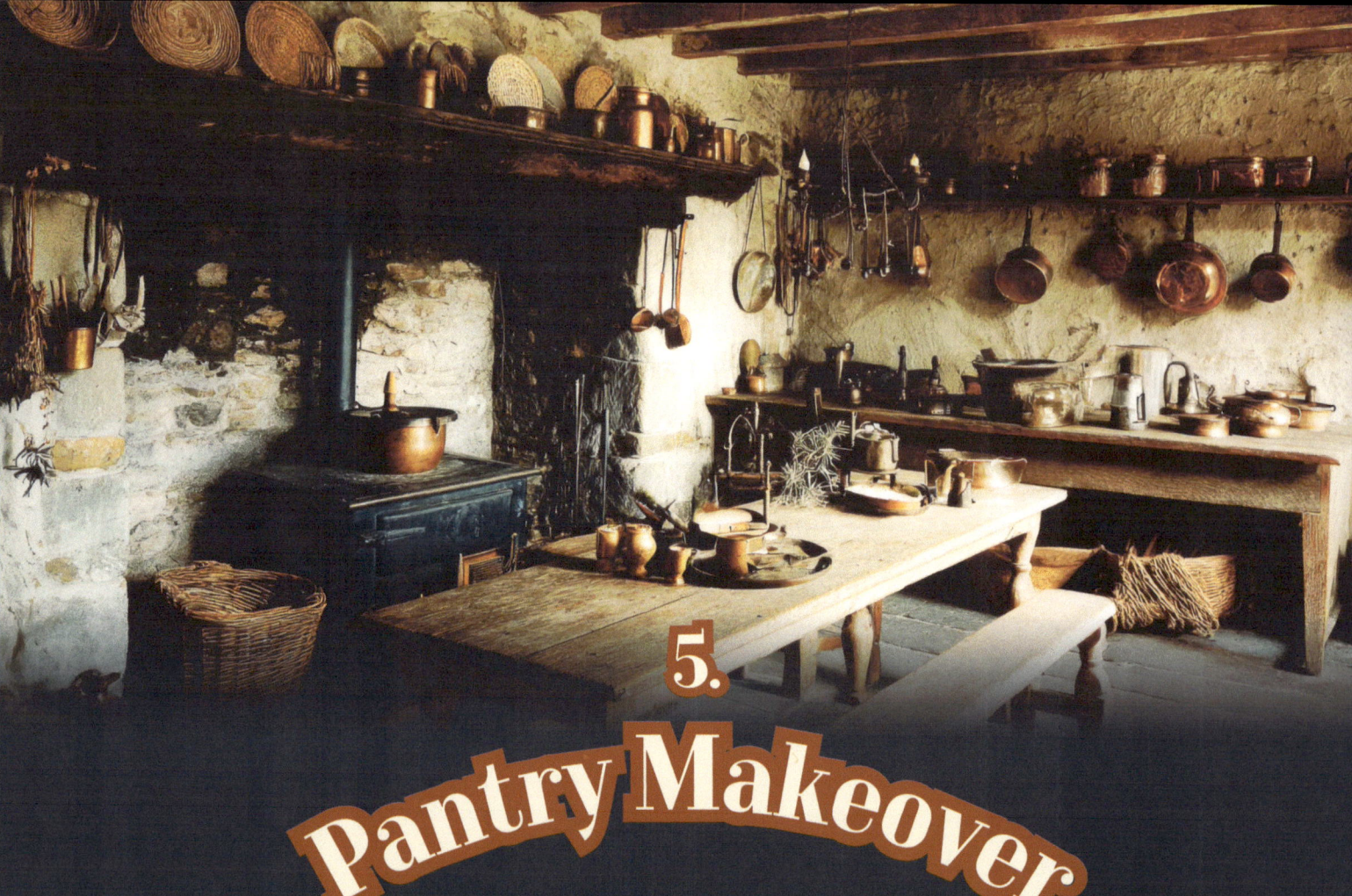

5.
Pantry Makeover

Spring crashes in like a lightning bolt, raw, unstoppable, charged with fresh possibility. It's the perfect spark to shake up your space and ignite real change where it counts most: your kitchen.

This is your call to action, to boldly clear out the hidden saboteurs lurking in your pantry: the processed snacks, artificial fillers, and tired habits that drain your energy. This isn't just tidying up; it's a powerful overhaul of how you fuel your life.

For me, this transformation didn't happen overnight. It took a full year of fierce dedication to morph my kitchen from a cluttered chaos of unhealthy snacks and quick fixes into a vibrant sanctuary pulsing with nourishment and life. Every shelf cleared, every fresh ingredient added, charged me with new vitality.

This journey demands grit and patience, a fearless commitment to change. But with every small victory, you'll feel momentum building, a surge of possibility that powers you onward. Let's take this leap together and turn your kitchen into a thriving heart of health and energy, lighting up your body, mind, and home.

Explore Your Kitchen

Each week, dive into your kitchen with intention, grab three items from your fridge and another three from your pantry. Don't just glance; really interrogate those labels. Notice how many ingredients you can pronounce without hesitation, and pay close attention to what's hiding in plain sight. Let curiosity lead you: research those mysterious names, uncover what fuels your body and what might be slowing you down. Short on time? No worries. Scale down the number of items; you're building awareness, not creating stress.

When shopping, zero in on three golden rules to keep your choices sharp and nourishing:

- **Ingredient Count:** Choose packages with five ingredients or fewer. Simplicity is your ally here; fewer components mean less processing and more real food.

- **Familiarity:** Reach for foods you can name without a dictionary. The familiar is usually free of sneaky additives and chemicals.

- **Vavor ingredients that feel alive:** Skip the neon colors and lab-made flavors-real nourishment doesn't need a costume.

Continue →

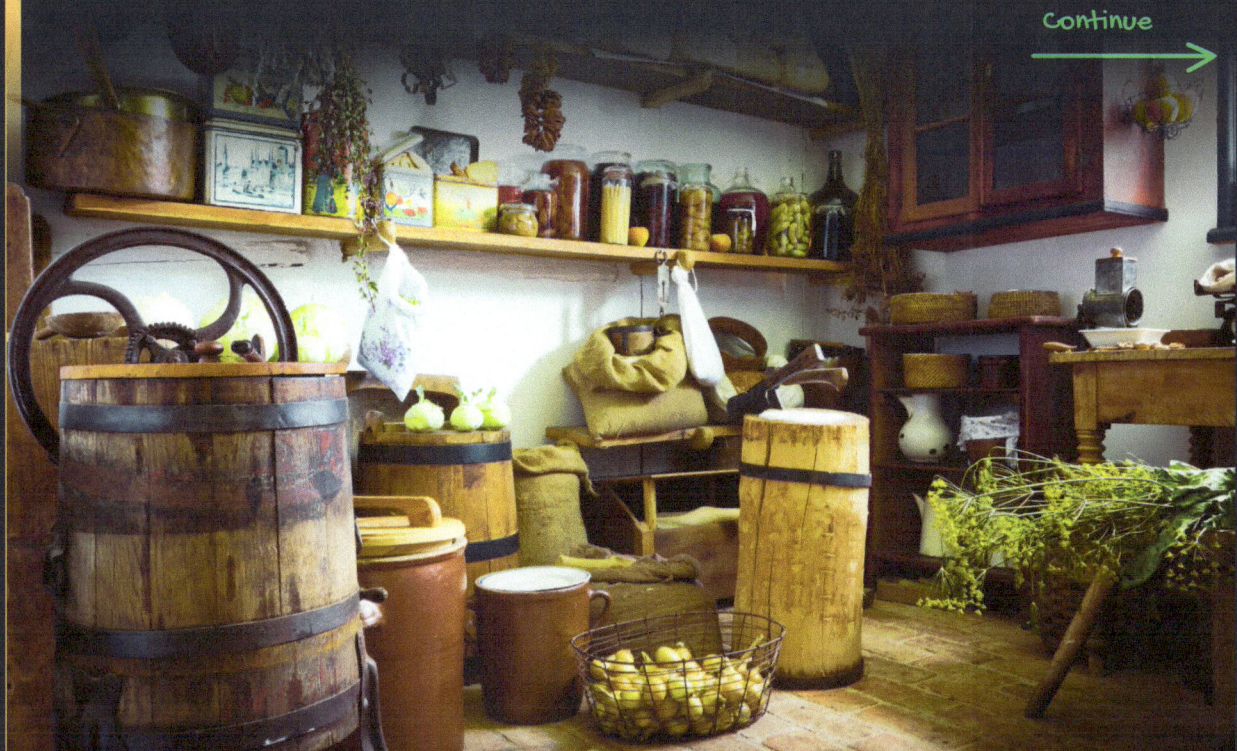

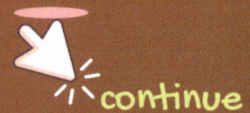
continue

Explore Your Kitchen

On a budget? Don't feel the pressure to toss what's already in your kitchen. Savor what you have. You can also gently weave in detoxifying teas or herbs I share in this book to support your body's natural reset. Meanwhile, step by step, start swapping out less nourishing items for vibrant, wholesome alternatives, or better yet, try crafting those foods from scratch to reconnect with the process.

Throughout this book, I'll share smart, inspiring ways to freeze select foods, methods designed to keep your kitchen a wellspring of vitality. Remember, transformation is a marathon, not a sprint. Your body deserves the time it needs to shed old habits and embrace a more vibrant, nourishing life. Trust the process, celebrate every small victory, and watch both your kitchen-and yourself-come alive with renewed energy.

Replacing Kitchen Essentials

Start by crafting your ultimate essentials list, a blueprint for the heart of your kitchen. With every grocery trip, swap out one or two items for clean, organic alternatives that elevate your food and your life. Here's a high-voltage guide to get you started, plus a few more powerhouse swaps to supercharge your pantry:

- Cooking Oil: Extra virgin olive or avocado oil
- Salt: Sea salt, Himalayan pink, or sun-dried rock salt
- Pepper: Whole peppercorns to grind fresh
- Spices: Organic and additive-free
- Flour: Organic wheat, almond, coconut, or stone-ground millet
- Baking Powder: Aluminum-free versions
- Beans: Dry beans for quality and control - try heirloom varieties like cranberry or black-eyed peas
- Tomato Sauce & Paste: Simple ingredients, organic if possible
- Herbs & Produce: Fresh, local, and organic when you can - honor bitter greens and wild herbs
- Sweeteners: Raw honey, maple syrup, coconut sugar
- Grains: Whole grains like quinoa and brown rice - include ancient grains like teff or sorghum
- Nut Butters: Pure nuts, no additives
- Condiments: Clean, simple ingredients only
- Vinegars: Raw apple cider, balsamic, or rice vinegar
- Dairy or Alternatives: Organic, unsweetened, and free of fillers - labneh, kefir, or coconut yogurt
- Broths & Stocks: Homemade or clean-label versions with real ingredients
- Extras: Black seeds (kalonji), dried barberries, saffron water, and roasted chickpeas—small touches, big legacy

Don't stress if you're on a budget, use what you have, and slowly shift toward healthier swaps. Every small change turns your kitchen into a vibrant, nourishing haven.

CRAFTING

Your Own Spices: *A CULINARY JOURNEY*

Investing in a high-quality spice grinder is not just a practical choice; it's a transformative step in elevating your culinary experience. By grinding your spices fresh, you can ensure that your spice jars are devoid of unnecessary additives and preservatives, all while capturing the deep, rich flavors that fresh spices offer. This process allows your dishes to truly shine, enhancing their complexity and aroma.

I personally find joy in using charming glass jars for my spice collection, taking the time to create customized labels that not only help with organization but also add a personal touch to my kitchen. Each jar tells a story of flavor and creativity.

The day I dedicate to grinding my spices often feels like a therapeutic practice. I remember moments from my childhood when my mom would ask me for a clean piece of paper. She would carefully fold it lengthwise, creating a makeshift funnel to transfer the freshly ground spices into our glass jars.

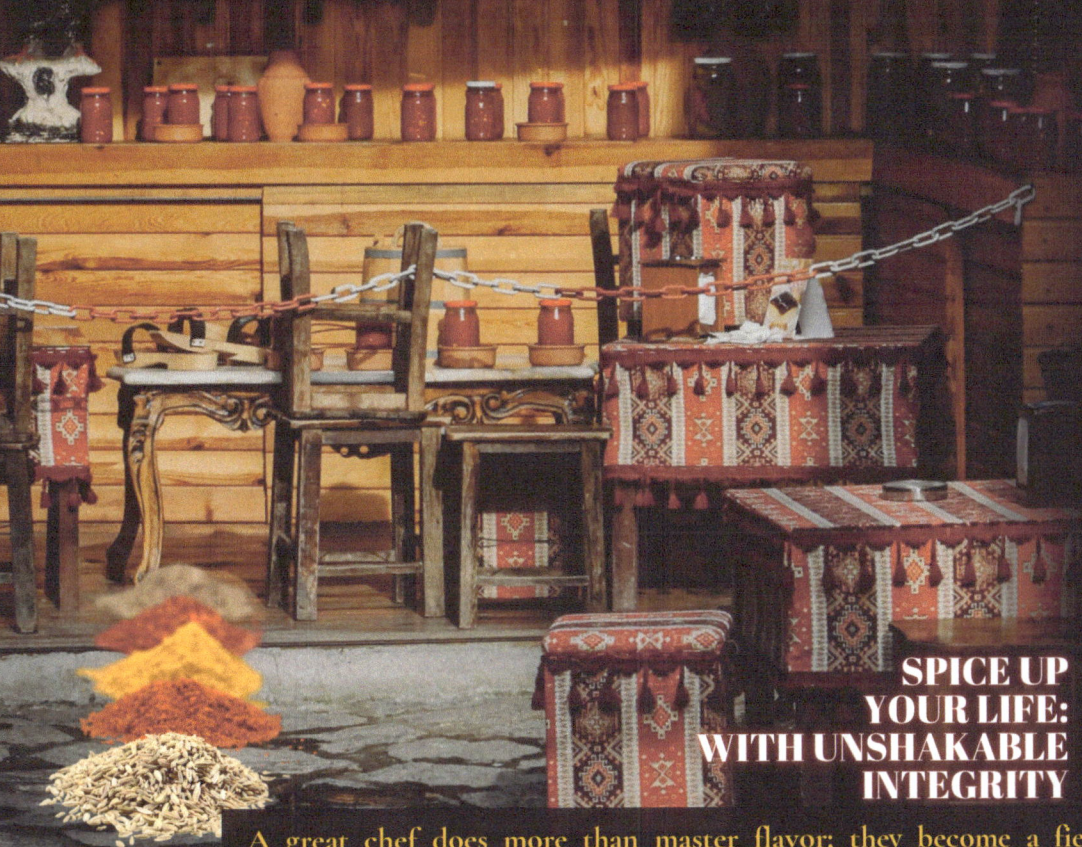

That simple yet ingenious method seemed magical, allowing us to reclaim every precious grain. These cherished memories spark creativity, lighting up the imaginative bulb in my mind and reminding me of the power of simplicity in the kitchen. Each grinding session is a celebration of flavor, nostalgia, and the endless possibilities that spices bring to our lives.

SPICE UP YOUR LIFE: WITH UNSHAKABLE INTEGRITY

A great chef does more than master flavor; they become a fierce guardian of ancient wisdom. Every spice carries a legacy, generations of stories, rituals, and purpose woven into each vibrant blend. When tossed carelessly, their soul fades; but with deliberate, reverent precision, they burst into brilliance.

True culinary magic isn't about domination; it's a symphony of harmony. The finest dishes honor their origins while boldly inviting fresh voices to the table. So season with courage, honor the craft that shaped these flavors, and let every pinch unleash the story it was born to tell, unfiltered, alive, and utterly unforgettable.

SAFFRON QUINOA & RHUBARB SKILLET CAKE

a warm dessert that tastes like resilience

INGREDIENTS

- 1 cup cooked quinoa (cooled)
- ½ cup almond flour
- 2 eggs or flax eggs
- 2 tbsp olive oil or melted ghee
- ¼ cup maple syrup or date syrup
- Pinch of saffron threads soaked in warm water
- ½ tsp cardamom
- 1 tsp baking powder
- 1 cup chopped fresh rhubarb
- Zest of one orange
- Crushed pistachios or sesame seeds for topping

INSTRUCTIONS:

- Preheat oven to 350°F (175°C).
- In a bowl, mix quinoa, almond flour, eggs, oil, syrup, saffron water, cardamom, and baking powder until smooth.
- Fold in rhubarb and orange zest.
- Pour into a greased skillet or baking dish.
- Top with crushed pistachios or sesame seeds.
- Bake for 25-30 minutes until golden and set.
- Serve warm, with yogurt or tahini drizzle if desired.

WHY IT HEALS:

Quinoa strengthens. Rhubarb clears. Saffron lifts the mood.
And baking, slow, fragrant, deliberate, reminds you that transformation takes heat.
This isn't just dessert. It's a way to soften what's been hardened.

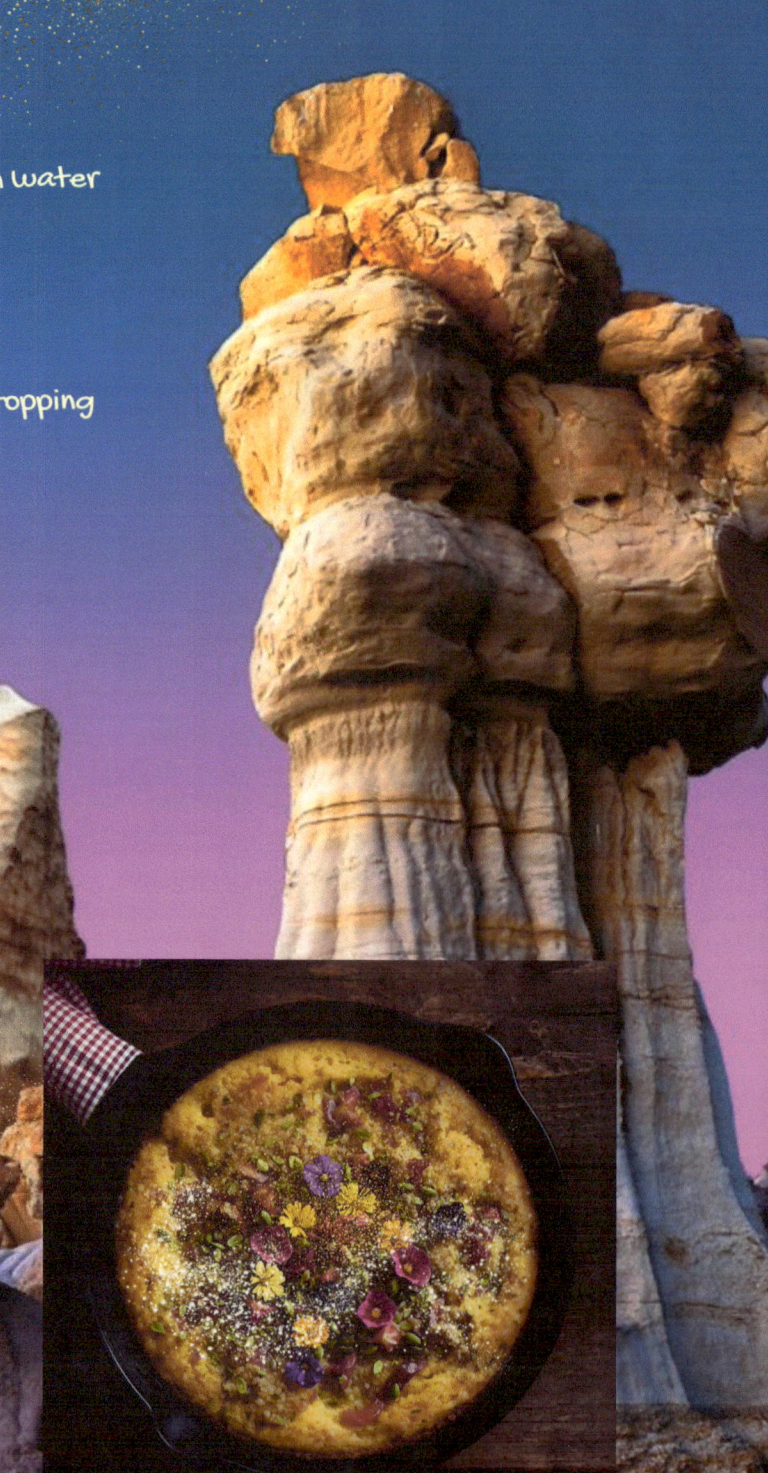

164

STONE-POT CHICKEN WITH BURNT DATES & BITTER GREENS

inspired by desert stews, ancestral fire, and the quiet strength of slow cooking

INGREDIENTS:

- Bone-in chicken thighs or lamb shanks
- Burnt onions (charred until blackened at the edges)
- Chopped bitter greens (like mustard, turnip, or fenugreek leaves)
- Dried dates (halved and lightly scorched in ghee)
- Crushed garlic
- Ground coriander, cumin, and black lime
- Sea salt
- Splash of vinegar or tamarind water
- Optional: saffron threads or dried rose petals for finish

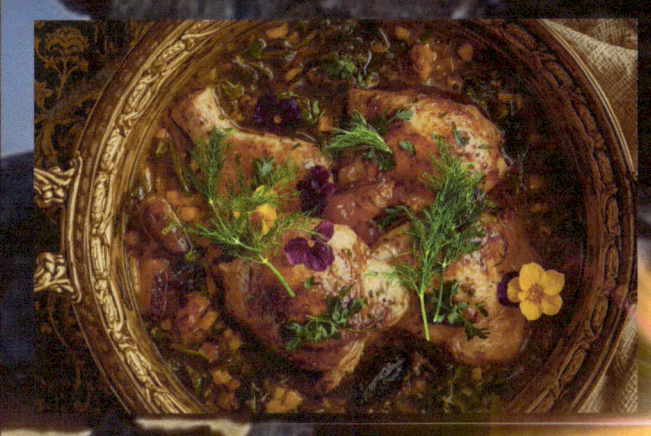

INSTRUCTIONS:

1. Start by browning the chicken or lamb well. Don't rush this part, get a nice color on the skin so it locks in all that flavor. You'll smell it when it's ready. Use a heavy pot if you have one; it holds heat better and cooks more evenly.

2. When the meat is browned, add the burnt onions and garlic. It might look a little blackened, but that's exactly what you want, it adds depth and a smoky warmth. Stir gently so you don't break everything apart.

3. Sprinkle in your spices, coriander, cumin, black lime, and stir them through. Let them wake up in the heat; you'll smell that fragrant mix almost immediately.

4. Pour in enough water to cover the meat, but don't flood the pot. You want a rich broth that's full of flavor, not soupy. Add the bitter greens and dates on top. Those greens might look tough, but they'll soften and add balance to all the richness.

5. Turn the heat down low and let it simmer. This is a slow process, so don't be tempted to check too often. Let the flavors mingle quietly for at least an hour and a half. The meat should become so tender it falls apart with just a touch of your fork.

6. Near the end, taste your broth and add a little vinegar or tamarind water if it needs brightness, this small step lifts everything. If you have saffron or rose petals, sprinkle them in now for that subtle finishing touch.

7. Serve this hearty stew hot, with flatbread to soak up every bit of the broth. Eat it slowly, savoring how each ingredient has softened and married over time.

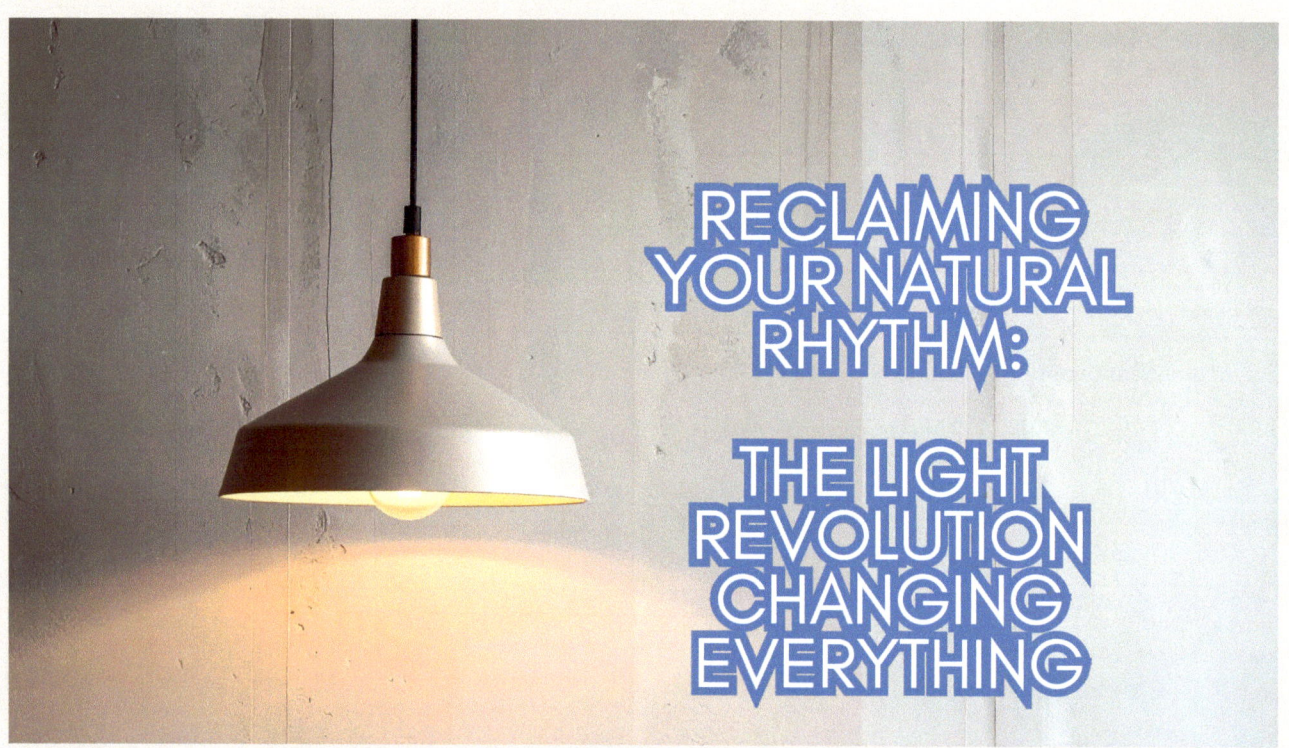

RECLAIMING YOUR NATURAL RHYTHM:

THE LIGHT REVOLUTION CHANGING EVERYTHING

In today's world, where screens glow endlessly and LED lights hum softly above us, we find ourselves submerged in artificial light, far removed from the sunlit rhythms that once governed human life. This isn't just a minor nuisance; it's a profound disruption. Our internal clocks, known as circadian rhythms, are finely tuned to the natural ebb and flow of daylight and darkness. These rhythms are essential not only for restful sleep but for orchestrating hormone production, metabolism, immune function, and even emotional well-being.

What's extraordinary -and still unfolding- is how much science has revealed about the deep impact of light on our biology. It turns out that typical indoor lighting provides only a fraction of the light intensity and spectrum our bodies depend on to stay synchronized. On a cloudy day, outdoor light delivers tens of thousands of lux, while the average indoor environment offers less than 150 lux, a staggering difference that leaves our biological clocks starving for proper signals.

The blue light emitted by screens and many artificial sources, while necessary for visibility, can overwhelm our eyes' ability to signal the brain when it's time to wind down. This suppresses melatonin, the hormone that triggers sleep, and delays the onset of rest. Research now shows that even brief evening exposure to artificial light can shift our sleep cycles by up to 90 minutes, disrupting the vital processes that repair and restore us overnight.

CONTINUE

Yet this disruption has a remarkable solution, one that is emerging at the cutting edge of health and technology. Innovations in wearable light therapy devices and circadian-friendly lighting are changing the game, allowing people to flood their systems with precisely the right wavelengths at the right times. Blue-light-blocking glasses with advanced filters, portable light visors delivering energizing doses of natural-spectrum light, and smart home lighting systems that adapt throughout the day are no longer futuristic ideas; they are becoming everyday tools for enhancing focus, mood, and sleep.

Alongside these technological advances, simple lifestyle shifts are proving incredibly powerful: stepping outside each morning to soak in natural sunlight, arranging workspaces near windows, and dimming lights as evening falls help reset and protect our internal clocks. The science is clear, realigning with natural light patterns can reduce risks of chronic disease, improve mental health, and dramatically boost energy and resilience.

This is not merely a new wellness trend. It is a profound shift in how we understand and nurture ourselves in an increasingly artificial world. The path forward is illuminated, not just by screens and bulbs, but by the ancient, life-affirming light of the sun. By consciously inviting natural light back into our lives, we reclaim balance, vitality, and a deep, sustaining connection to the rhythms that have shaped humanity from the very beginning.

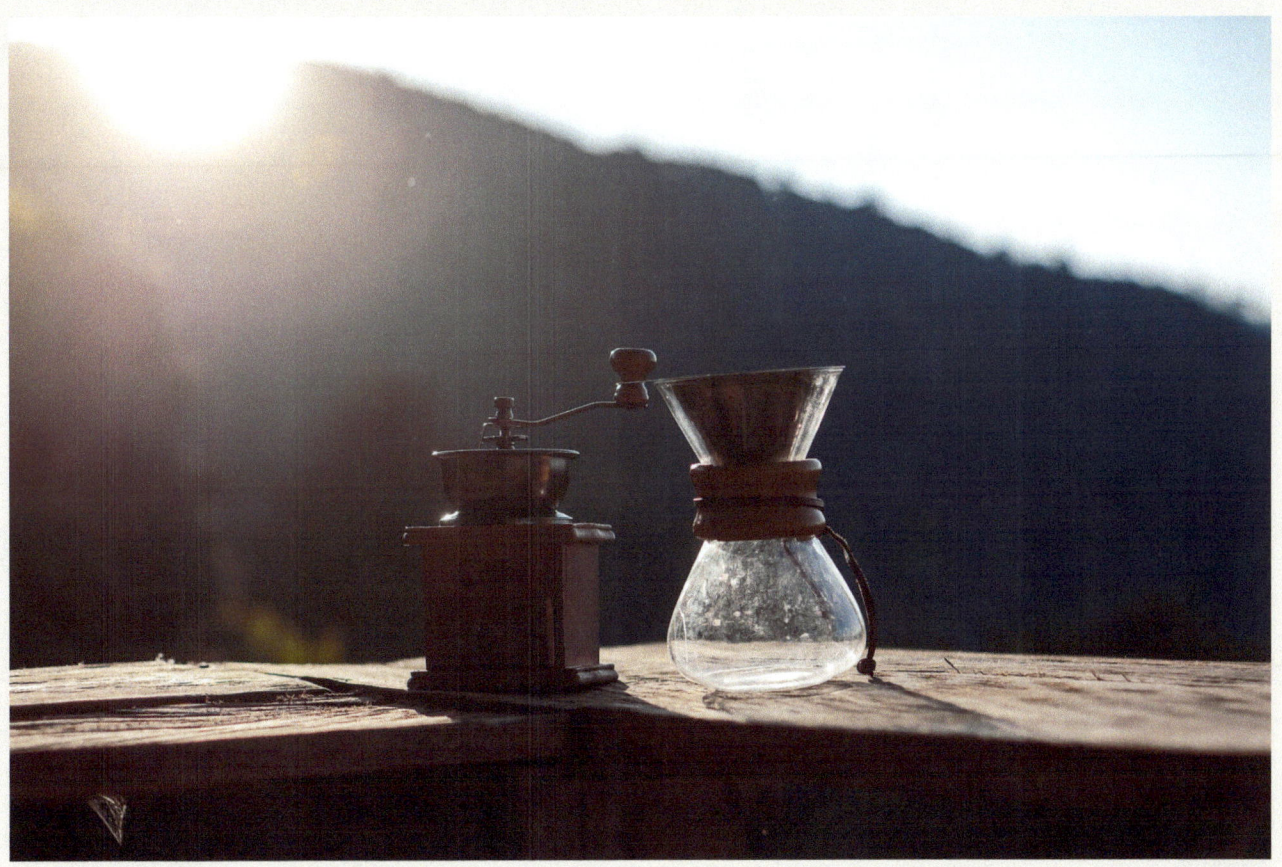

Vegan Mortadella with Rose and Smoke
THE ORCHARD'S BREATH

BASE (SILKY EMULSION)
- Protein: Cooked chickpeas + steamed vital wheat gluten (for structure)
- Binder: Silken tofu + olive oil (mimics the creamy fat pockets)
- Texture dots: Whole pistachios + soaked barberries (zereshk)
- Seasoning: White pepper, coriander, cumin, garlic, a touch of nutmeg

UZBEK-PERSIAN INFUSION
- Saffron water: Bloomed threads folded into the mix for golden warmth
- Rose petals: Finely ground, for perfume and subtle floral lift
- Pomegranate molasses: A spoonful in the blend for tang and depth
- Optional: Dried apricot powder or grated carrot for a sweet, orchard-like undertone

TECHNIQUE
1. Blend chickpeas, tofu, oil, and spices into a smooth paste.
2. Fold in vital wheat gluten until it forms a pliable dough. Add pistachios + barberries.
3. Shape into a log, wrap tightly in parchment + foil (or muslin for a rustic look).
4. Steam for 1.5-2 hours until firm and sliceable.
5. Smoke gently (cold-smoke or quick hot-smoke) with apricot or mulberry wood. Toss in dried orange peel or green tea leaves for a wellness-forward aromatic smoke.

SERVING
- Slice thin, serve with fresh herbs (sabzi khordan), radishes, and warm bread.
- A drizzle of honey-free glaze (pomegranate molasses + date syrup + lemon) makes it jewel-like and vegan-friendly.

WHY IT WORKS
- Nourishment with lightness: Chickpeas, tofu, and gluten create strength without burden, satisfying yet airy, like a meal that steadies rather than weighs.

- Echoes of ancestry: Saffron, rose, pistachio, barberry, and apricot smoke carry the voices of Persian gardens and Uzbek orchards, binding the present to the past.
- Charm of smoke: A handful of tea leaves or citrus peel turns cooking into ceremony, a small act of alchemy that perfumes the air as much as the food.
- Jewels within: Pistachios and barberries scatter through the loaf like confetti in rice, a reminder that beauty belongs inside the body as much as on the table.

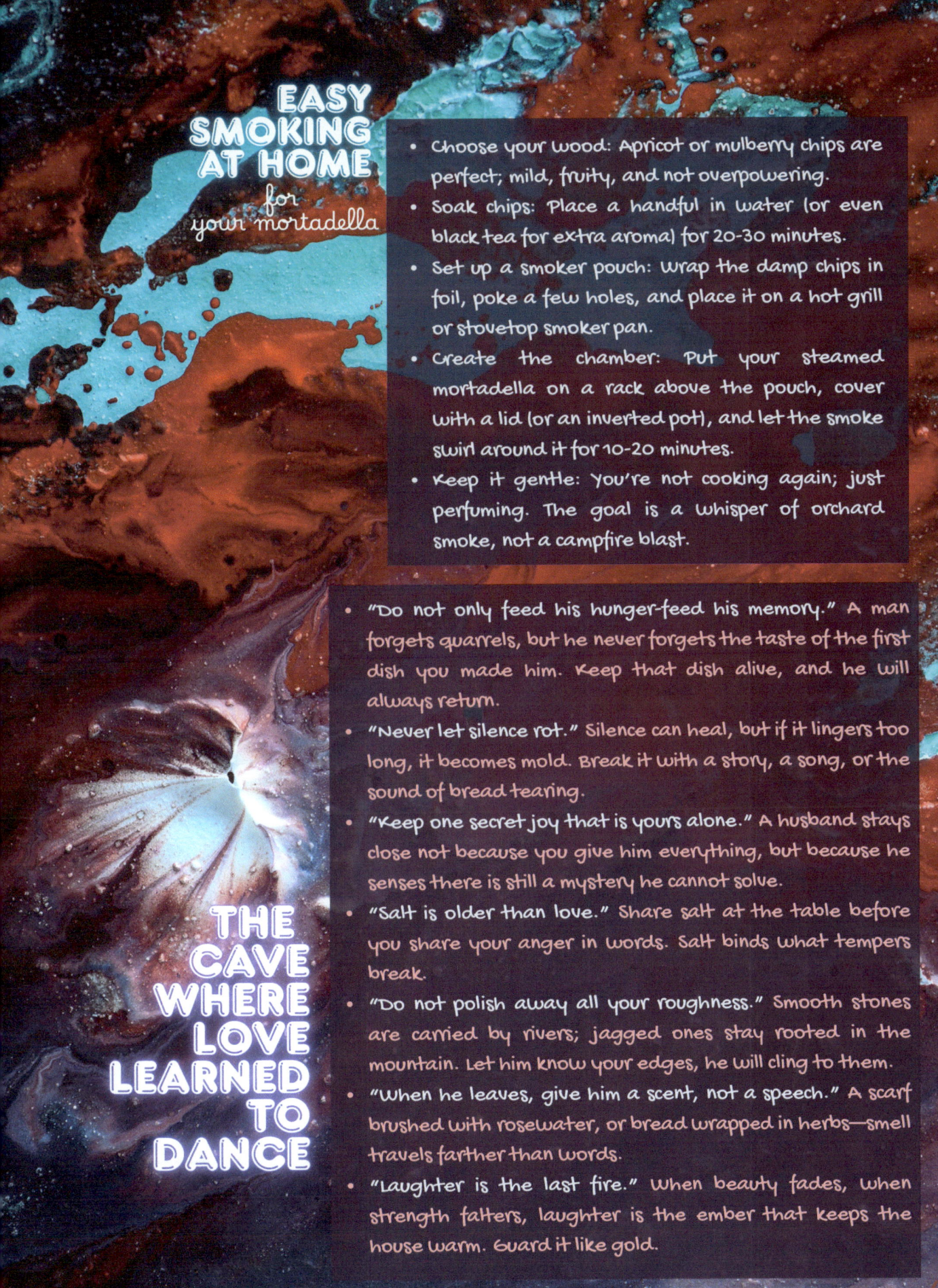

EASY SMOKING AT HOME
for your mortadella

- Choose your wood: Apricot or mulberry chips are perfect; mild, fruity, and not overpowering.
- Soak chips: Place a handful in water (or even black tea for extra aroma) for 20-30 minutes.
- Set up a smoker pouch: Wrap the damp chips in foil, poke a few holes, and place it on a hot grill or stovetop smoker pan.
- Create the chamber: Put your steamed mortadella on a rack above the pouch, cover with a lid (or an inverted pot), and let the smoke swirl around it for 10-20 minutes.
- Keep it gentle: You're not cooking again; just perfuming. The goal is a whisper of orchard smoke, not a campfire blast.

THE CAVE WHERE LOVE LEARNED TO DANCE

- "Do not only feed his hunger-feed his memory." A man forgets quarrels, but he never forgets the taste of the first dish you made him. Keep that dish alive, and he will always return.
- "Never let silence rot." Silence can heal, but if it lingers too long, it becomes mold. Break it with a story, a song, or the sound of bread tearing.
- "Keep one secret joy that is yours alone." A husband stays close not because you give him everything, but because he senses there is still a mystery he cannot solve.
- "Salt is older than love." Share salt at the table before you share your anger in words. Salt binds what tempers break.
- "Do not polish away all your roughness." Smooth stones are carried by rivers; jagged ones stay rooted in the mountain. Let him know your edges, he will cling to them.
- "When he leaves, give him a scent, not a speech." A scarf brushed with rosewater, or bread wrapped in herbs—smell travels farther than words.
- "Laughter is the last fire." When beauty fades, when strength falters, laughter is the ember that keeps the house warm. Guard it like gold.

Apple Cider Vinegar:
The Shot That Broke the Chains

I never thought I'd say this, but I owe my sanity to apple cider vinegar.

For years, my nights were a battlefield. The migraines came like storms-merciless, mind-splitting pain that drove me into a dark room where even breathing felt too loud. I'd curl up in silence, clutching a bottle of painkillers, swallowing six at a time just to make it through. Looking back, I wonder if the headaches were only half the enemy... and the pills themselves had become the other chain, tightening around me with every dose.

Then one night, in a moment of sheer desperation, I reached for something different. A bottle of apple cider vinegar. I took a raw shot, no water, no honey, just fire. It burned all the way down, and then something extraordinary happened. Within minutes, the pain dissolved. Not dulled.... gone.

I tried it again the next time, and again after that. Within days, the migraines vanished. And with them, so did my dependence on the pills.

Was it the vinegar healing my headaches? Was it breaking an addiction I didn't even realize had me by the throat? Maybe both. All I know is that I walked out of that darkness free.

And here's what makes it even more astonishing: apple cider vinegar isn't just folklore. Research shows it can help regulate blood sugar, improve insulin sensitivity, and even curb appetite, powerful shifts that ripple through the body's systems. Its natural compounds fight inflammation, support immunity, and may influence the very pathways tied to pain and cravings.

For me, it wasn't just a remedy; it was redemption. A humble bottle became the key that unlocked my freedom. And every time I see it now, I remember those nights in the dark, the pills lined up on the nightstand, and the moment I finally broke the chains.

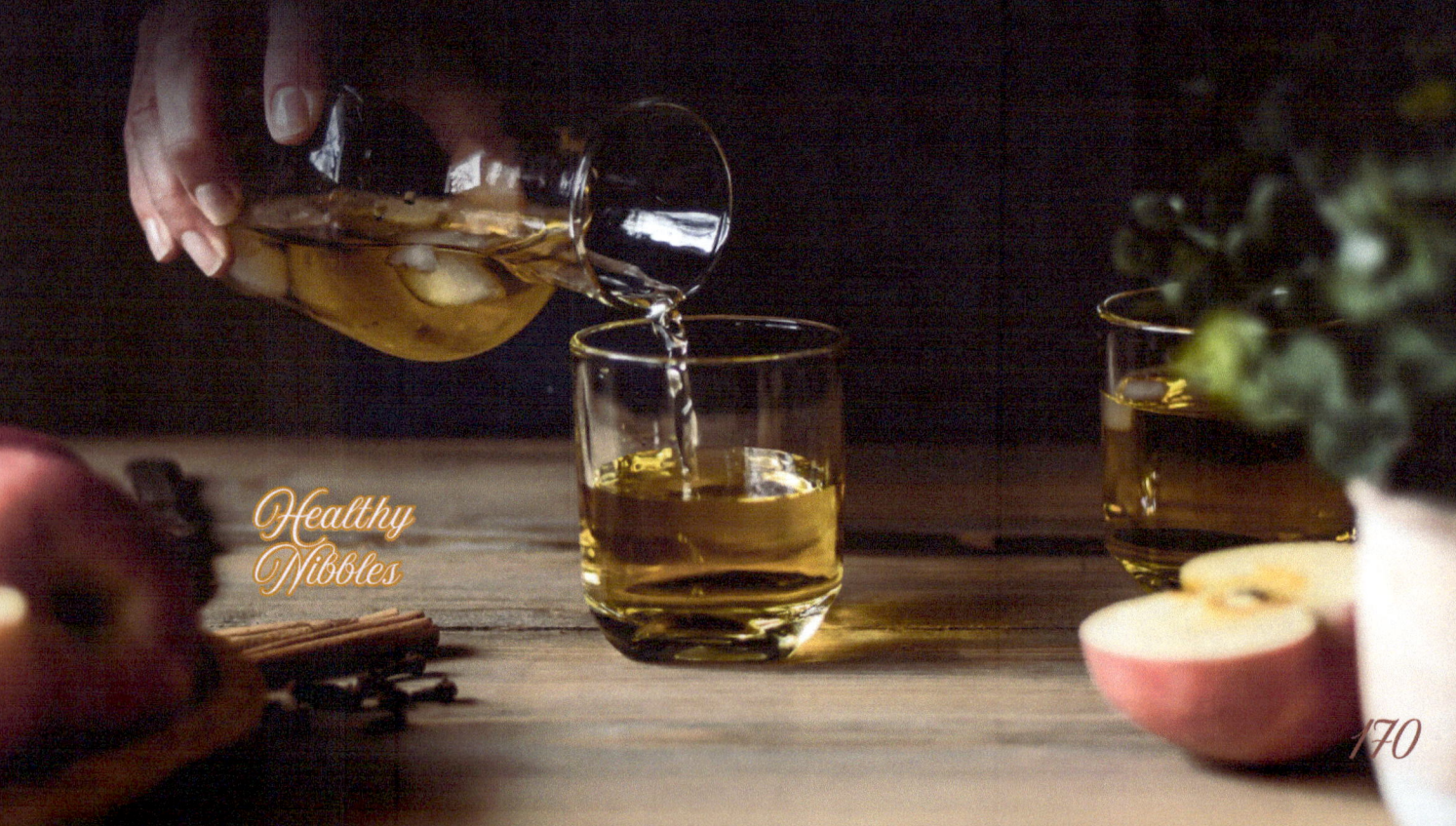

Healthy Nibbles

Wild Blueberries

Move over, gummy bears—this year's real candy lives in the freezer aisle. Organic wild blueberries are tiny bursts of joy, packed with antioxidants, fiber, and vitamin C. They fuel gut health, strengthen immunity, calm inflammation, protect the heart, and even sharpen memory. Sure, you can toss them into smoothies, but here's my favorite trick: roll the frozen berries in a squeeze of lemon and a dusting of coconut sugar, and suddenly they're tangy, sparkling little jewels. Cold, sour-sweet, and electric on the tongue, they're nature's candy, and they've officially earned the title: Candy of the Year!

Sea Moss:
Ageless Glam from the Sea

It's almost tragic how often we ignore nature's treasures until our bodies demand attention. For me, it was the drag of iodine deficiency; fatigue so heavy it dulled my sparkle, a metabolism slowed to a crawl. Then came sea moss, the ocean's own beauty elixir. Rich in iodine, it revived my thyroid, restored my energy, and brought me back to life.

But the true surprise? The glow. Sea moss, loaded with antioxidants and over ninety minerals, worked like nature's collagen, smoothing, hydrating, and giving my skin a luminous, ageless radiance. This wasn't just health; it was glam. A secret that nourishes from within, strengthens immunity, and leaves you glowing like you've stepped off a runway.

Sea moss isn't a trend, it's timeless. A beauty ally, a wellness powerhouse, and the ultimate reminder that agelessness isn't about chasing youth, it's about feeding your body what it craves to shine

Papaya:

Growing up, papaya was a rare jewel I never encountered. It wasn't until I moved to the US that I first laid eyes on this tropical treasure. Its glowing orange flesh looked like a gemstone split open, and the first taste, sweet, sun-kissed, with whispers of melon and peach, was like biting into a sunset. I was instantly enchanted.

From that moment, papaya became more than a fruit; it became a symbol of discovery, of savoring beauty in unexpected places. And beyond its allure, papaya is a true powerhouse: aiding digestion with its natural enzymes, draping the skin in a radiant glow, fortifying immunity, and protecting vision with its vibrant nutrients. Rich in vitamin C, fiber, folate, and vitamin A, it's both nourishment and luxury.

To me, papaya isn't just food; it's edible glamour, a reminder that wellness can taste like paradise

Legacy Isn't Always a Group Project

It started with a plate, something sweet, golden, sliced just right. The kind of offering that looks innocent until you remember the history behind it. In certain circles, apologies don't come with words. They come with fruit. Or favors. Or a sudden invitation after seasons of silence. You learn to read between the gestures.

I grew up believing that closeness meant safety. That being surrounded by voices, by footsteps, by shared meals, was the secret to a long, vibrant life. And science backs it up: people who live among others, who share space and stories, tend to live longer, heal faster, and carry joy like a birthright. I built my world around that idea. My work celebrates it.

But here's the twist no one warned me about: proximity doesn't always mean protection. Sometimes, the very people who shaped your early laughter become the ones who sharpen your silence.

In my culture, connection is sacred, but also theatrical. We don't do quiet disappointment. We do opera. Someone might ignore you for a decade, then show up at your celebration with a gift and a grudge. Another might bless you with one hand and curse your ambition with the other. There's love, yes, but it's often tangled in hierarchy, jealousy, and the kind of emotional debt that accrues interest.

I tried. I tolerated. I hosted dinners where I cooked with my heart and cried in the pantry. I answered calls that drained me, attended gatherings that felt like auditions, and smiled through stories that erased me. I thought endurance was loyalty. I thought silence was strength.
Then came the mango. And the realization that I was allergic; not to the fruit, but to the performance.
Still, I gave chances. I showed up. I offered grace where I should've drawn a line. I told myself that misunderstanding was part of the dance, that maybe they didn't mean it, maybe they didn't know better, maybe love just looked different here.

But eventually, I realized: I was shrinking to fit a mold I'd already outgrown.

So I did something unexpected. I chose peace over performance. I reimagined connection, not as obligation, but as alignment. I began to gather with those who saw me clearly, who didn't flinch at my truth or compete with my joy. I built a new kind of closeness, one rooted in mutual respect, not shared history.

And yes, I still believe in togetherness. I still adore the idea of a home filled with laughter, layered stories, and the kind of warmth that lingers. But now I know: longevity isn't just about who's around you, it's about how you feel when you're with them.

It's about whether your presence feels like permission or performance. Whether your joy is welcomed or weighed. I began to notice the difference between being included and being seen. Between being tolerated and being treasured. And once you taste that kind of clarity, you can't go back to pretending.

Healing meant rewriting the rules. It meant honoring the beauty without reenacting the pain. It meant giving chances, yes, but also recognizing when those chances become cycles. Above all, it meant telling the truth, not just the polished parts, but the raw, radiant middle. In these pages, closeness is redefined. Not as obligation, but as nourishment. Not as performance, but as peace. And sometimes, the most courageous act is choosing what sustains the soul, even if it looks like distance. This isn't abandonment. It's return. To self. To clarity. To a kind of love that doesn't require shrinking.

The Conscience That Doesn't Flinch

There's a moment after harm, after the sting, the silence, the spiral, when my conscience wakes up. Not gently. It barges in, pushy and uninvited, dragging clarity behind it like a suitcase full of truths I wasn't ready to unpack.

I resist it at first. I'm tired. I want rest, not reckoning. But my conscience doesn't care for timing. It speaks in questions I'd rather not answer. What if it wasn't malice, but circumstance? What if the mistreatment was a symptom, not a sentence? What if love, in its flawed dialect, was trying to speak?

I hate how it makes me think. But I respect it. Because even when I'm bruised, my conscience refuses to let bitterness build a home. It rinses my heart just enough to keep it soft. Not naïve, just open.

And so, I hand healing to time. I let time do its slow, sacred work. I don't chase closure anymore. I don't audition for reconciliation. I simply wait. If my conscience was right, the rivers will join. If not, I'll still be whole; no longer shrinking, no longer performing, no longer mistaking endurance for love.

This is not forgetting. It's remembering differently. It's choosing peace without erasing the past. It's honoring the ache without reenacting the opera. It's knowing that sometimes, the most radical act of love is distance. And sometimes, the most honest kind of closeness is the one that begins with solitude.

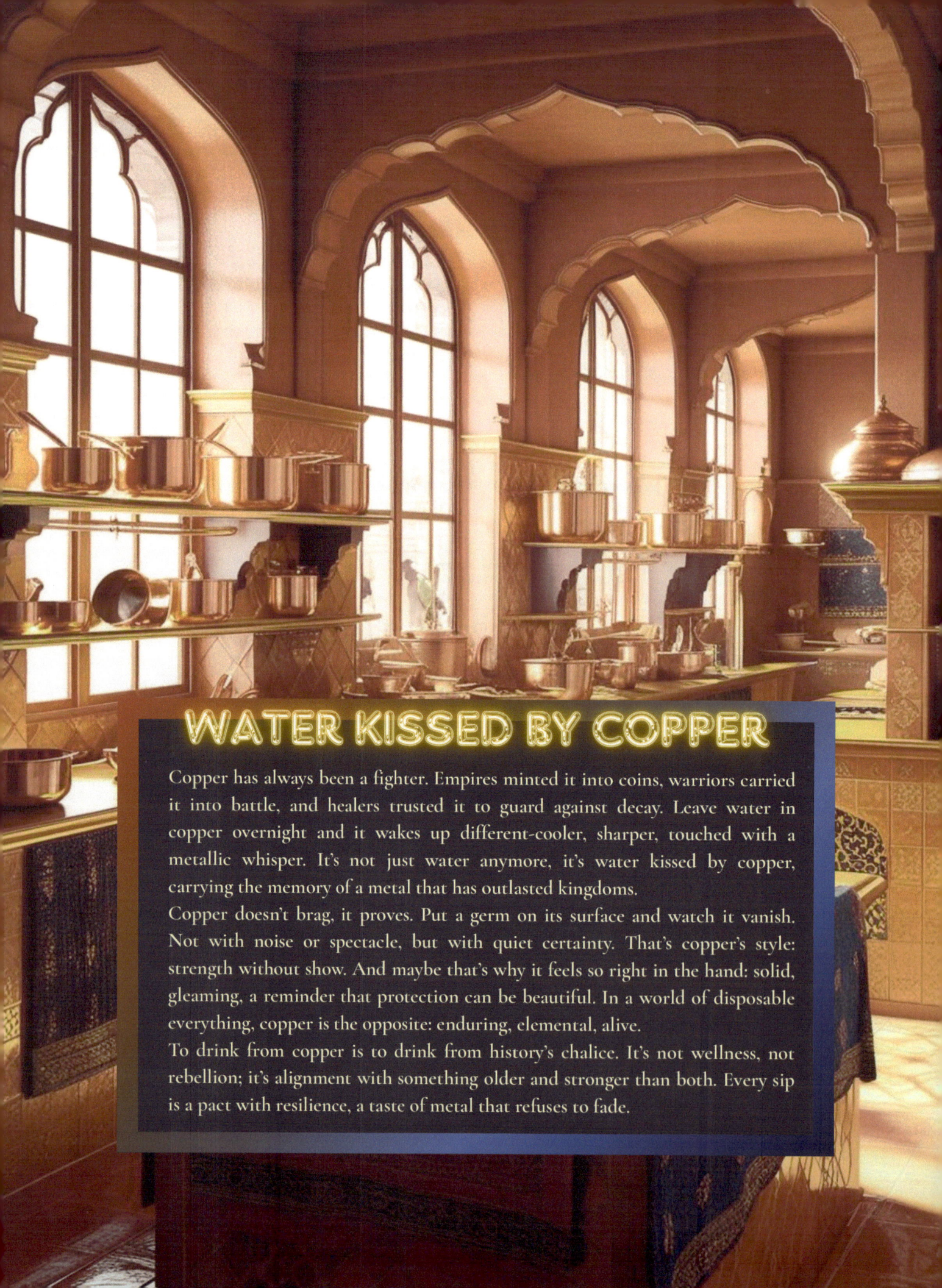

WATER KISSED BY COPPER

Copper has always been a fighter. Empires minted it into coins, warriors carried it into battle, and healers trusted it to guard against decay. Leave water in copper overnight and it wakes up different-cooler, sharper, touched with a metallic whisper. It's not just water anymore, it's water kissed by copper, carrying the memory of a metal that has outlasted kingdoms.

Copper doesn't brag, it proves. Put a germ on its surface and watch it vanish. Not with noise or spectacle, but with quiet certainty. That's copper's style: strength without show. And maybe that's why it feels so right in the hand: solid, gleaming, a reminder that protection can be beautiful. In a world of disposable everything, copper is the opposite: enduring, elemental, alive.

To drink from copper is to drink from history's chalice. It's not wellness, not rebellion; it's alignment with something older and stronger than both. Every sip is a pact with resilience, a taste of metal that refuses to fade.

HAZARDOUS OILS: A CLOSER LOOK AT SEED OILS

For years I trusted the tidy promises on the label: heart-healthy, neutral, vegetable-based. I welcomed corn and canola into my kitchen like quiet allies. Then my body spoke in a language I could not ignore-skin that swelled, features that softened into someone else's face, a persistent fog that felt like betrayal. The culprit was not glamour or stress. It was the bottle on my shelf.

The Chemistry That Quietly Undermines You

• Heat and chemistry change the fat
Extreme heat and aggressive solvents rearrange fatty acids, producing oxidized lipids and trans-type isomers. These altered molecules do not behave like whole-food fats; they trigger inflammation and cellular stress over time.

• Aldehydes and reactive compounds
When degraded oils reach cooking temperatures, they emit reactive compounds that burden detox systems and inflame tissues. This is not immediate drama; it's a slow accumulation that rewrites how cells respond to stress.

• Stripped of protection
Refining strips away antioxidants, micronutrients, and phytonutrients that normally temper fat's reactivity. What you're left with is an oil that can oxidize easily and has nothing to protect your cells from that damage.

How This Shows Up in Life

. Skin - Puffiness, persistent redness, slow-healing rashes, new sensitivities after meals.
Why it matters: oxidized fats generate inflammatory signals that alter skin barrier function and immune reactivity. These aren't cosmetic annoyances; they're visible evidence of systemic oxidative stress.

• Energy - Midday crashes, prolonged recovery after exertion, an ongoing low-level fatigue that coffee won't fix.
Why it matters: damaged lipids interfere with cellular respiration and mitochondrial efficiency, turning steady energy into repeated burnout.

• Metabolism - Weight plateaus or slow, stubborn gain despite "doing the work."
Why it matters: trans-like isomers and oxidized fats disrupt lipid metabolism and insulin signaling, quietly favoring fat storage and metabolic dysregulation over time.

• Cardiovascular signals - Elevated resting heart sensations, poor circulation, or family-history markers that suddenly feel closer.
Why it matters: trans fats and oxidized lipids promote arterial inflammation, raise LDL, and lower HDL-small daily exposures compound into a measurable cardiovascular risk.

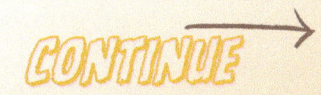
CONTINUE →

. **Digestion - Bloating, gas, slowed digestion, or new intolerance to previously comfortable foods.**
Why it matters: damaged fats alter gut microbiome balance and intestinal lining resilience, producing chronic low-grade inflammation and barrier permeability.

• **Cognition and Mood - Brain fog, increased anxiety, dulled focus, mood swings after processed-food meals.**
Why it matters: lipid oxidation products cross the blood—brain barrier and provoke neuroinflammation, which shows up as cognitive fuzz and emotional volatility.

• **Immune and Recovery - Longer healing times, flares of autoimmune-like symptoms, greater post-illness exhaustion.**
Why it matters: persistent oxidative stress and inflammatory signaling impair immune regulation and tissue repair.

• **Subclinical damage adds up - No dramatic hospital moment. Just accrual.**
Why it matters: small molecular insults from daily cooking oils accumulate silently for years; they show up later as chronic disease markers rather than an overnight emergency.

Hidden Places RBD Oils Hide

- Salad dressings and mayonnaise
- Packaged baked goods and crackers
- Snack foods, chips, and fries
- Margarine and spreads
- Ready-made sauces and condiments
- Some boxed or canned goods that list "vegetable oil" without specificity

If a product lists "vegetable oil" or "partially hydrogenated oil," assume it's industrial seed oil unless otherwise specified.

Quick Pantry Scanner Checklist

- Read the label: If it says "vegetable oil" without specificity, skip it.
- Avoid "partially hydrogenated": That signals industrial trans fats.
- Look for processing words: Refined, bleached, deodorized, hexane-extracted.
- Prefer named oils: If a label names olive, avocado, or sesame and lists minimal processing, it's usually better.
- Check ingredient count: Fewer, recognizable ingredients win.
- Note placement: Ingredients high on the list mean more of that ingredient per serving.

The Rise of Real Oils:
A Revolution in Every Drop

The oils you choose matter; they shape the flavor, nutrition, and quality of every meal. Switching to high-quality oils can elevate both taste and health, making every dish a step toward better well-being.

High-Heat Cooking

For frying, sautéing, and roasting, select oils that hold their integrity under high temperatures:

- Avocado Oil: Rich in monounsaturated fats and boasts a high smoke point, perfect for searing meats and vegetables.
- Coconut Oil: Packed with medium-chain triglycerides, adding depth to Asian-inspired dishes and baked goods.
- Ghee: A clarified butter with a nutty, luxurious taste, free from lactose and loaded with beneficial compounds.

Low-Heat Cooking

For gentle cooking and finishing touches, opt for oils that shine in their raw form:

Extra Virgin Olive Oil: A powerhouse of antioxidants and rich flavor, best for dressings, drizzling, or light sautéing.

The Power of Cold-Pressed Oils

Minimal processing preserves nutrients, antioxidants, and purity, ensuring better absorption, better health, and better taste.

Every meal is an opportunity for transformation. why settle for less when the revolution has already begun?

The Luxe Glow of Power Naps

Sleep has always felt like my most cherished embrace; a sacred time where my body is cradled in care, floating effortlessly toward renewal. It's the pause my soul longs for, the perfect retreat from the endless hum of thoughts that fill my waking hours.

And then, there are mornings, those glorious first moments when the air feels velvet-soft, the sky stretches in quiet elegance, and I rise feeling light, refreshed, limitless. There's something undeniably divine about starting the day with a heart full of possibility, as if I'm stepping into a world that's designed just for me.

By midday, the pull of rest calls again, a gentle invitation to drift, recharge, and surrender. I welcome it, whether for a brief escape or a deep, luxurious reset that cocoons me in stillness. Those longer naps? Pure devotion, a stolen moment where the world pauses and I emerge, revived, luminous, gloriously untouchable.

Waking is no less exquisite. I rise feeling weightless, as if the universe has handed me a second sunrise, a brand-new beginning to step forward with grace and ease. Sleep is not just an escape; it is my greatest indulgence, my softest luxury, my forever love.

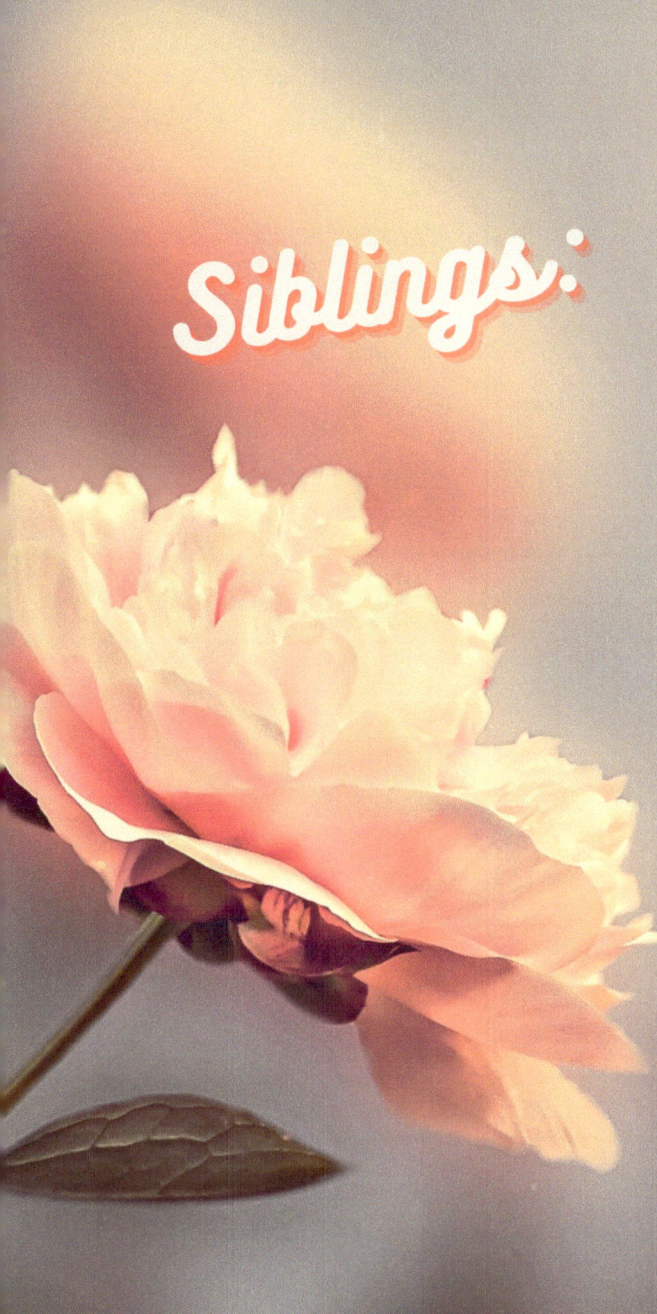

Siblings:

Siblings, the quiet, unwavering constellations in the galaxy of our lives. The ones who walk beside us from the very first steps, the ones who know our joys and sorrows without a single word spoken. To have a sister or a brother is to hold a rare and precious gift, a love so lavishly etched into the essence of our existence that it defies explanation. They are our true soulmates.

I remember, as a child, watching that sentimental movie, the one where lost siblings find their way back to each other through a song their mother once sang. And me, the eldest, full of hope and intention, wanted to teach my own siblings a song, a safeguard against life's uncertainties, a melody to anchor us, no matter where life pulled us.

My bond with them is stitched with a kind of parental devotion, an unshakable instinct to protect, guide, and always be there. And why? Because I am blessed beyond words to have siblings who respond to the smallest whisper of my need. Who, when I utter a quiet "ouch," come running before the echo fades.
I remember that frigid winter night, stranded, out of gas, uncertain who to turn to. Of all the people I could call, I chose my little sister, who was an hour away. And without hesitation, she simply said, "I'm on my way."

Siblings, the bond that no storm can break, no distance can erode, no quarrel can truly shake. It's a privilege, a luxury, an inheritance of love. I think back to the darkest day of my life, watching my daughter undergo surgery, and still, I see them—my siblings, beside me from dawn until midnight, their eyes filled with quiet sorrow, holding back tears so I wouldn't have to shed mine alone.

Siblings are irreplaceable. They are the diamonds in the depths of my heart, shining with a light that time, grief, and life's trials will never dim. IA

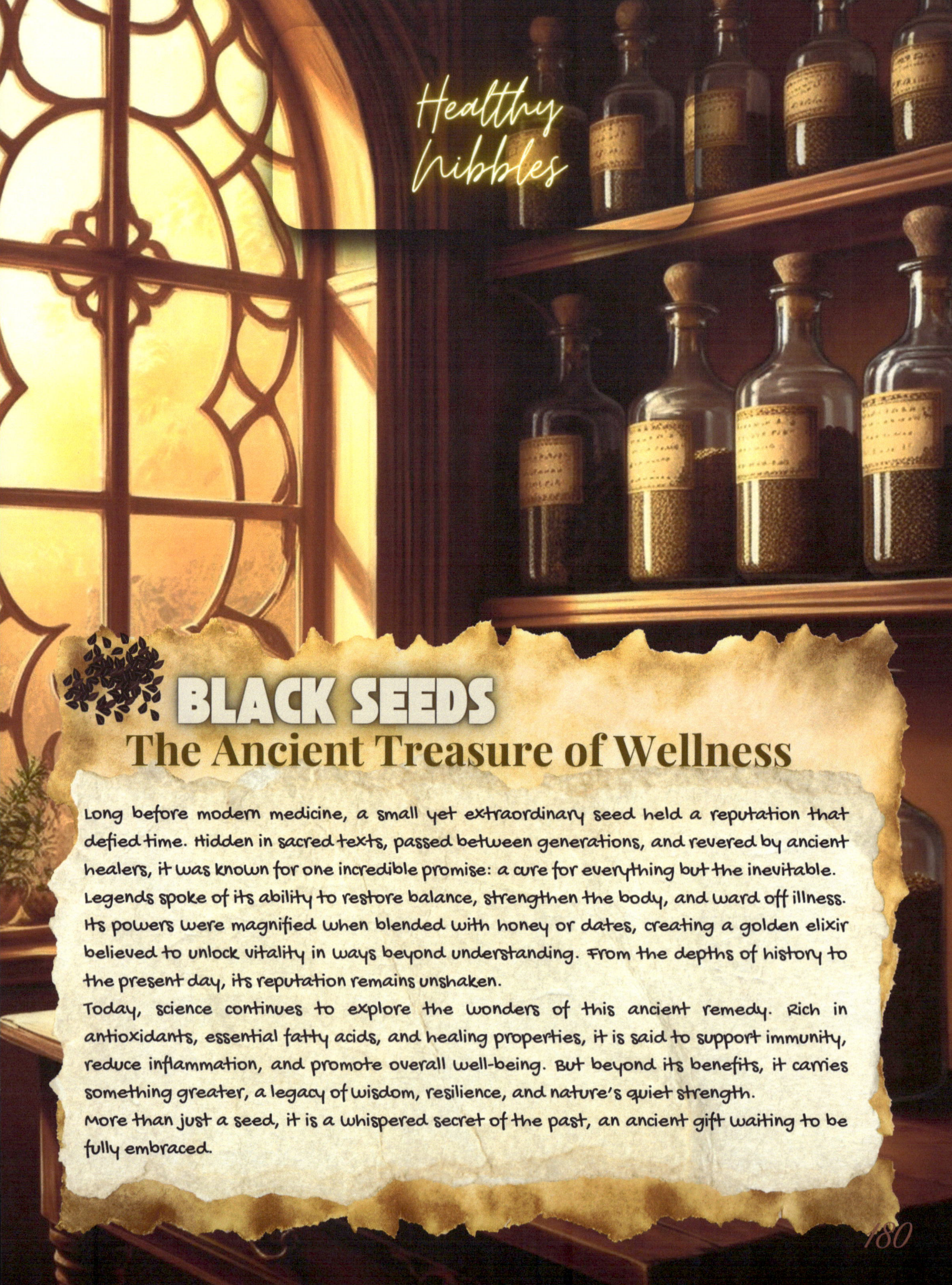

BLACK SEEDS
The Ancient Treasure of Wellness

Long before modern medicine, a small yet extraordinary seed held a reputation that defied time. Hidden in sacred texts, passed between generations, and revered by ancient healers, it was known for one incredible promise: a cure for everything but the inevitable. Legends spoke of its ability to restore balance, strengthen the body, and ward off illness. Its powers were magnified when blended with honey or dates, creating a golden elixir believed to unlock vitality in ways beyond understanding. From the depths of history to the present day, its reputation remains unshaken.

Today, science continues to explore the wonders of this ancient remedy. Rich in antioxidants, essential fatty acids, and healing properties, it is said to support immunity, reduce inflammation, and promote overall well-being. But beyond its benefits, it carries something greater, a legacy of wisdom, resilience, and nature's quiet strength.

More than just a seed, it is a whispered secret of the past, an ancient gift waiting to be fully embraced.

CHICKPEAS:

I cook them in big batches (pressure cooker, no fuss), then let them become what they want to be. Sometimes that means roasting them until golden and crisp, tossed with rosemary, thyme, and a whisper of smoked paprika. A snack with crunch and soul.

Other days, it's hummus: creamy, cold, kissed with garlic and lemon. I blend in ice for silkiness, then dip with carrots and celery, the kind of snack that feels like care.
When I want comfort, I mash chickpeas with a spoonful of mayo, lemon, and salt. Tucked into a wrap with fresh veggies, it's simple, satisfying, quietly nostalgic.

But my favorite chickpea memory isn't from a kitchen; it's from the street. I was little, and the vendor would scoop steaming chickpeas into a paper cup, then pile on pickled red radish, cumin, hot sauce, brown vinegar, and soft chunks of boiled potato. The smell hit first, spicy, sour, earthy, and I'd clutch that cup like treasure. My mom didn't approve; she worried about street germs. So I'd rope my aunt into taking me, both of us pretending it was just a walk. But we knew what we were after. That snack was messy and bold, and it made me feel alive. We'd eat it standing up, sauce dripping, laughing at nothing in particular. It wasn't fancy, but it was everything.

BEYOND FLAVOR, CHICKPEAS ARE PURE NOURISHMENT.

They're packed with plant-based protein and fiber, which help you feel full longer and support digestion. They're gentle on blood sugar, making them a smart choice for steady energy. Chickpeas also help lower cholesterol, which supports heart health. Mineral-wise, they're rich in iron, magnesium, and phosphorus, essential for energy, bone strength, and overall vitality. And they're a great source of folate, a B vitamin that supports cell repair and DNA synthesis.

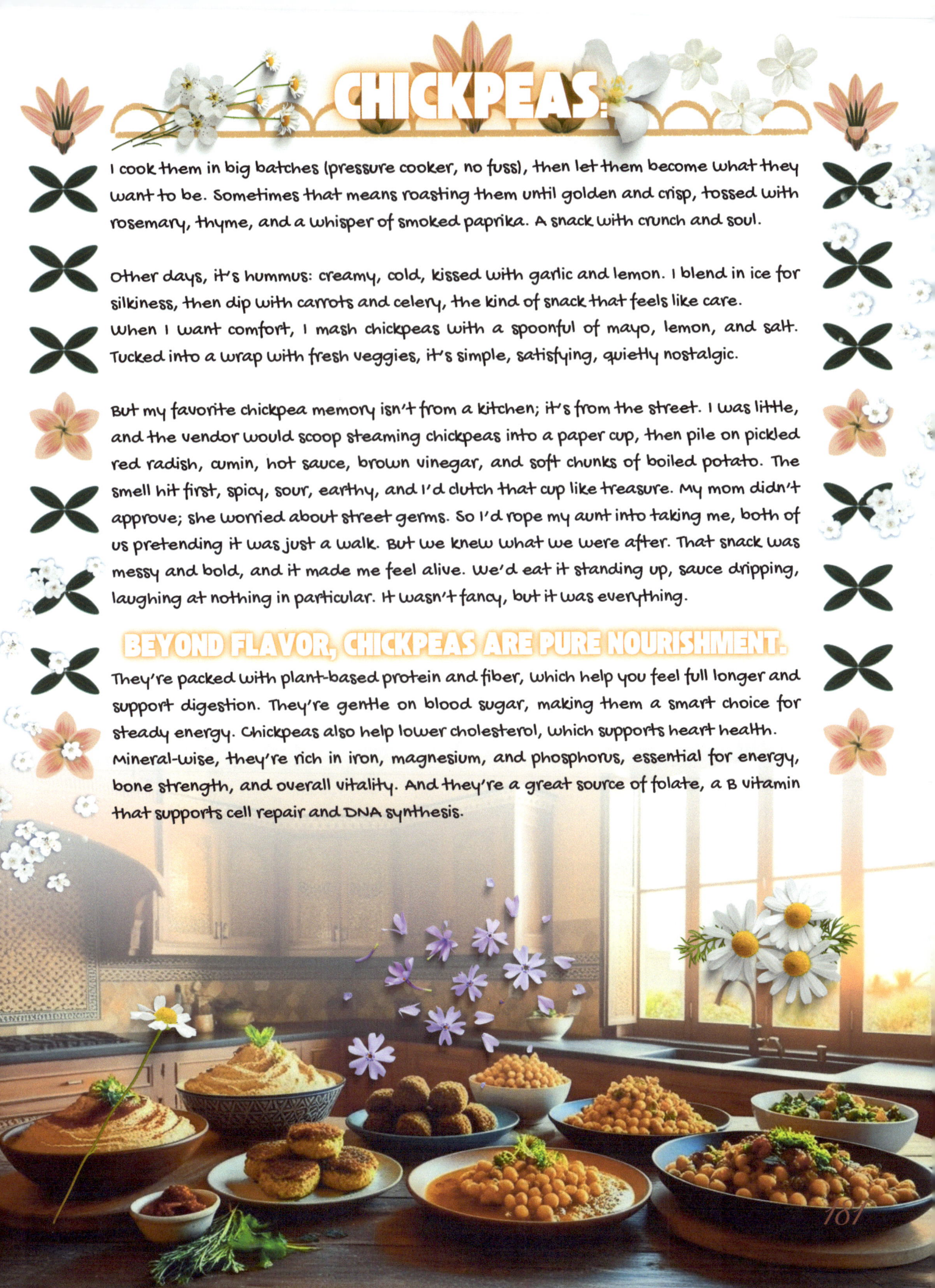

SHOOR NAKHUT:
THE FINAL GATHERING OF SPRING

Shoor nakhut, a typical dish of Uzbek cuisine, is more than just a recipe; it's a symbol of hospitality and festivity that marks the beginning of any gathering. I can hardly recall a time when I prepared it solely for my family; it's always been a staple reserved for celebrations and communal feasts. At these vibrant events, the competition among the ladies to create the most exquisite version of shoor nakhut is fierce, each cook adding her unique touch and quiet brilliance. It's not just about impressing, it's about being seen. About showing what you carry, what you've inherited, and what you dare to reimagine. That's why this dish belongs here, at the end. It holds the spirit this book has been simmering toward: generous, bold, and rooted in something deeper than instruction.

Throughout my culinary journey, I've made a remarkable discovery that I believe will redefine shoor nakhut as we know it. This innovative approach enhances the flavor profile while maintaining the dish's traditional charm, ensuring that every bite resonates with the rich heritage of Uzbek cuisine. But it's more than a technique, it's a quiet reclamation. A final gesture. A reminder that tradition isn't sacred because it's untouched, but because it survives transformation. This version carries my story, my season, and maybe yours too. Let it be the dish that says: you've arrived. And you're ready to serve something only you could make.

INGREDIENTS:

- 5 cups of cooked chickpeas (including 1 cup of their cooking liquid for added flavor and moisture)
- 5 tablespoons of avocado oil - 1 yellow onion, thinly sliced (for sweetness and depth of flavor)
- 3 tablespoons minced garlic
- 1 tablespoon homemade garam masala (or store-bought) warming
- ½ teaspoon turmeric, vibrant
- 2 teaspoons ground cumin, earthy
- 1 teaspoon ground coriander, citrusy undertone
- Salt and freshly ground black pepper, to taste
- 2 bay leaves, depth
- A dash of cayenne pepper powder, heat
- 1 tablespoon organic vegetable bouillon paste
- ½ cup of organic ketchup
- 1 jar of pickled vegetables, including the liquid
- ¼ to ½ cup of organic white vinegar
- A few tablespoons of your favorite cayenne pepper hot sauce

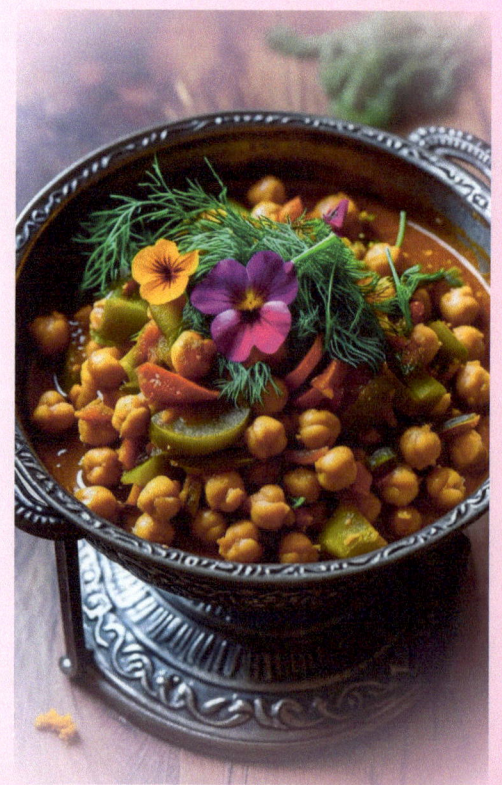

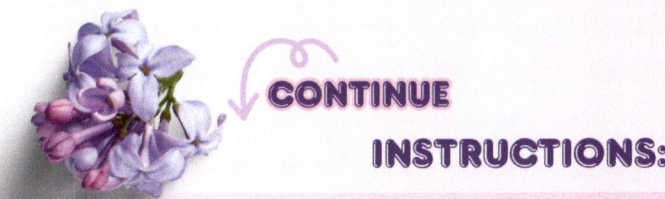

CONTINUE

INSTRUCTIONS:

1. Begin by preheating a large, deep stainless steel pan over medium heat. Once the pan is hot, carefully add the avocado oil and allow it to heat for about 30 seconds until shimmering, but not smoking.

2. Introduce the thinly sliced onion to the pan, stirring frequently. Your goal is to caramelize the onions to a rich golden brown without venturing into over-browning territory, which could impart a burnt flavor. This process typically takes about 8-10 minutes.

3. Next, add the minced garlic along with the garam masala, turmeric, cumin, coriander, salt, and pepper. Stir this aromatic mixture for roughly 30 seconds to release the spices' fragrance, ensuring the garlic does not burn.

4. Pour in the organic ketchup and vegetable bouillon paste, stirring to combine all ingredients. Continue to cook on medium-low heat for a few minutes, allowing the flavors to meld together beautifully.

5. Carefully add the cooked chickpeas along with their reserved liquid, the pickled vegetables, and the white vinegar. Gently bring this mixture to a boil while stirring cautiously to prevent breaking the chickpeas. Focus on your movements and maintain a positive spirit, as love is indeed the most essential ingredient in any dish.

6. Once boiling, reduce the heat to low and let the mixture simmer for about 5 minutes, allowing the flavors to develop. During the last minute of cooking, incorporate your preferred amount of cayenne pepper hot sauce.

7. To serve, remove from heat and garnish with a sprinkle of dried dill, a dusting of cumin, and a sprinkle of sumac for a burst of color and flavor.

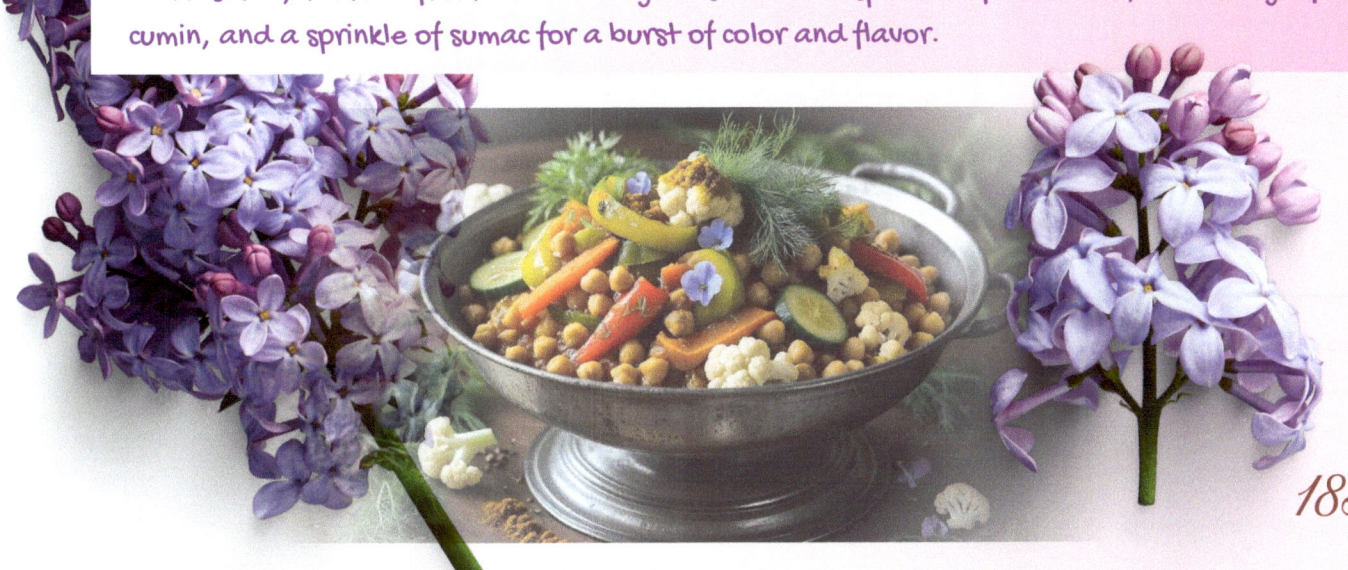

This book is a slow simmer,

low heat, gentle pace, step by step.

I want you to experience each recipe through the eyes of a beginner,

because that's exactly how I learned to cook, through stories,

mistakes, and the occasional culinary disaster.

Cooking isn't just about following instructions; it's about feeling the

process, embracing errors, and learning as you go. My first 'fancy' meal after

moving in with my husband? An impressively burnt chicken, a true

masterpiece of charred perfection. He was kind

enough to eat it anyway!

And that's the heart of this book.

I want you to grow alongside me, not by copying, but by exploring,

discovering, and celebrating your own small victories.

Let each chapter unfold at its own pace,

slow, thoughtful, full of love.

There's more heat and shedding ahead, when you're ready, the next season

will rise to meet you.